LOVE SONGS TO MY BRAIN

LOVE SONGS TO MY BRAIN

David Joel Orenstein

Copyright © 2019, David Joel Orenstein
All rights reserved
Cover art and design by Shirin Raban
Print layout by Booknook.biz

CONTENTS

EMERGENCE	1
COMPUTERIZED AXIAL TOMOGRAPHY ONE	15
DREAMING AN IMMACULATE CRANIOTOMY	24
NEUROLOGY 101	27
AMBULANCE TO ADULTHOOD	31
DECEMBER 19, 1979	34
TEN DAYS	45
THE MAN IN THE INTENSIVE CARE UNIT	51
HOMECOMING	54
THE NIGHTMARE	63
BACK TO SCHOOL	67
CRIES AND PANGS OF THE BODYMIND	73
WELCOME TO MIGRAINEVILLE	80
TONIC - CLONIC	87
MERRITT AND PUTNAM'S DILANTIN ISLAND	93
COMPUTERIZED AXIAL TOMOGRAPHY TWO	96
RADIATION WILL MAKE YOU LIKE NEW	98
SUSIE AT THE EPICENTER OF BUDDING LOVE AND BRAIN CANCER	102
COMPUTERIZED AXIAL TOMOGRAPHY THREE	105
COMPUTERIZED AXIAL TOMOGRAPHY FOUR	106

LIKE DOLPHINS	107
THIS IS HOW I SEE THE WORLD	110
AUDITORY ISOLATION: THIS IS HOW I HEAR THE WORLD	118
MULTITASKING	125
MEMORIES OF MEMORY	127
THE HOT HEAD	129
THE UNCLE HARRY SYNDROME	133
BIRTH OF AN EMPATH	136
MIGRAINE: MY WORLD AND WELCOME TO IT	139
LOVE IS AN OPIUM POPPY	149
LOVE IN A TIME OF POST TRAUMATIC STRESS	162
GLIOBLASTOMA MULTIFORM STAGE FOUR	165
RIVERS AND DAMS	166
MIGRAINE AS A VOICE	171
THE SOUNDS OF MADNESS	174
TWO FRIENDS, MY DOCTOR AND YOSEMITE	177
SHERPAS OF THE MIND	180
THE PRACTICE MEANS PRACTICE	191
THE GRATITUDE WINDOW	196
A FANCIFUL CONVERSATION WITH THE MINISTER OF MIGRAINE AURAS AND HEADACHES	201
THE BIRTHDAY PRESENT	218
SURVIVORS AND COMPANIONS	220
DER MENSCH TRACHT UND GOTT LACHT	222
ACKNOWLEDGEMENTS	225

EMERGENCE

November 1979
the weekend begins
afternoon sun hanging low
on those darkening autumn days

a mischievous boy
rebellious troublemaker
attention-seeking clown

emerging from adolescence
each department falling into place
school
jobs
girls
self-confidence
athletic dreams
unruly hair

the mazik
slowly becoming
a mensch

the mail brings more brochures
colleges that like my SAT scores

and eagerly awaited letters
from the girls I met last summer

the adolescent has had a romance
with a creative college junior
she said
someday you'll know who you are

but the boy still wants
to play with his friends
flatulence and fast cars

once I said to myself
I'm in love with
the internal combustion engine

one of those letters
is inviting me to Susie's prom!

another girl signs off
I love you
loves me!

I wander around the house
in a daze
like Charlie Brown
getting that note
from the little red-haired girl

I'm just getting started

Ken led me to AP classes
and despite myself
I scored five in history

I can compete
with the smart kids
maybe college is not so daunting
I can adapt
learn how to learn

today I'm reading about Raskolnikov
the cop knows he did it

I don't need to cram forty books into my brain
choose a few
enjoy them without indigestion
and regurgitate
my dawning penetrating literary acumen
on the AP in May

John arrives in the afternoon
his '66 Pontiac Tempest
recently mag wheeled
turbo mufflered
a new 400 cubic inch engine

I put Raskolnikov away
the Tempest is fast
but my obsession with cars is flaming out

besides I have become a runner
when the others are exhausted
I keep running

when I am exhausted
I keep running
I can push myself

Blake and Dave call me
the Gazelle
but I'm too lazy to join the track team

cruising in the thundering Pontiac
through November's long shadows
wind blowing through my curls
towards Cal State Northridge
my default college
for Crosby Stills and Nash tickets

the Beatles speak to me
illuminating life
rearranging my intracranial connections

growing up on Penny Lane
faces I remember
the eyes in which I'll see nothing

but CSN's syrupy harmonies
are the soundtrack
to last summer's
leadership camp love fest
and to these final months of high school

we sang CSN
over the campfire
the girls resting their heads on my lap
something about those cheesy lyrics

becoming oneself
saying goodbye to the past

meshing with the freedom
excitement and bittersweetness
of growing up

I am floating through these last months
floating as the Tempest parks aside the expansive lawn
at Cal State N

the afternoon air
cool and pleasant
I am growing comfortable
in my skin

cruising the metamorphosis
from boy to man

having been a sad bully
tormenting the weaker boys
and that sweet girl
with myoclonic seizures

the leadership training camp
launched my rehabilitation

arriving quiet
unsure of my status
watching the cool kids
choose a nebbish to pounce on
tormenting him with their creative gifts

I watched
from the unanticipated mantle
of being popular

shuddering
and tossing
that out forever

stepping out of the Tempest
into the cool afternoon air
the future school beckons me
but the expansive lawn
looks slightly skewed

I say to John
I'm getting old
I need glasses

we buy the tickets
and head home
towards the darkening western sky

at Shabbat dinner I say
make an appointment with an optometrist

from my parents
I expect a practical response
but Mom is startled

the boys and I see a movie
Yanks and Commies sharing missiles
destroying an Earth killing meteor
another fable depicting the cold war's demise

once home I watch
Ted Koppel's show
The Iran Crisis: America Held Hostage

dismissing my vision's as of yet
mild malfunction
I go to my parking attendant job the next evening

how I love this play work
how I love bragging about it
the BMW's
the Porsche 911s
the tips we're supposed to turn in
the gourmet food we're fed as scraps
having helped Farrah Fawcett from her 450SL
and taken her Benz for a ride
top down
through the Santa Monica mountains
the wind blowing through my hair

driving home from work
the freeway lights
appear distorted

the next morning my head aches
Dad takes me to Kaiser

you have double vision I'm told
could be a cluster headache
what's that?
a type of migraine

fulfilling my expectation
doc writes prescription
and says
If this doesn't work
we'll know to look for something else

his remark evaporates
I just want my pills
which work like a charm

amusing myself with the mild diplopia
my family proceeds to a restaurant
I have my first French dip sandwich

prompt resolution of the headache
dinner with my family
I'm feeling euphoric

yes
things are falling into place
I've stopped tormenting my sister
getting along with Mom and Dad

soon off to D.C.
with tickets to see summer camp friends
and the White House

after graduation
a year abroad with new friends
a springboard for entry into the world
and how I'm going to change it

in bed
however
I am overcome by panic
I haven't thought about college
I haven't thought about the future

a major?
the right school?
a career?

I had
an unrealistic fantasy
of being an airline pilot
dismissed by my parents with
a knowing silence

friends have been visiting colleges
my head has been in Car and Driver magazine

yes I've done some work
but I still want to play

from my nightstand I grab that pile
of unread brochures
nervously perusing the schools' faculty lists
majors and minors
and find something to hold on to

college: Such and Such University
major: international relations
career: I'll save the world

my future solved
panic subsides
I sink beneath the blankets
thankful for the pills
thankful for my family
thankful for my warm bed
and for this cozy middle-class house
sheltering me as December approaches

I drift off to sleep
deep euphoric sleep

I wake up
Monday morning
there is double vision
headache
nausea
no school for me today

Mom takes me to Kaiser
we see an urgent care doctor

who sends us to an ophthalmologist
who sends us to a neurologist

with headache
lack of appetite
and a strange
unfamiliar feeling
soon to be labeled
Lethargy

I just want to return to bed
after swallowing the pill
that will rid me of this
pesky infection

I have never seen a neurologist
this is major league medicine
why am I here

the pediatrician I had seen
now and then
saw my sore throats
and broken bones
wrote prescriptions
sent me to the basement to have casts set

Mom scolding me
do you know how much
each one of those X-rays costs

I also
preferred avoiding him

and those yearly examinations
of testicular development

now I walk into something new
a neurologist
a woman
young and attractive
a sharp dresser
with long brown hair
and sexy boots climbing up her long legs

my head aches
my eyes aren't working correctly
tired listless and getting scared
but those horny synapses keep firing

she says
look left and right
up and down
close your eyes
touch your nose
smile
show your teeth
walk in a straight line
heel to toe

shining a flashlight
into my eyes
her eyes
looking for something

I take note of her diploma
doctor of neurology
an accomplishment

she is at the forefront
of medicine
of the advance of women

my head hurts
the world looks slightly askew
I am tired and want to go to sleep
she schedules a CAT scan
a what?

something about more detailed pictures
putting your head in a washing machine
they are new
comes here once a week
in a van

be here on Wednesday

weary and listless
aching head
two of everything

everyone I see
has a conjoined twin

I step into the van
housing this new technology

my head resting on the plastic board
not comfortable
but not painful

a swirling noisy machine
yes, like inside a washing machine

then to the waiting room
lethargic
I haven't been eating or drinking
my head hurts
Mom is with me
I don't say anything
no magazine reading
I just sit there

every few minutes
the intercom calls
Dr. Campofiori please, Dr. Campofiori

who is Dr. Campofiori
and why do they keep calling him
Dr. Campfiori, please, Dr. Campofiori

COMPUTERIZED AXIAL TOMOGRAPHY ONE

name: David Orenstein
date of birth: 18 May 1962
date of exam: 5 December 1979

Report: There is a mass lesion in the region of the central median nucleus of the thalamus on the left which enhances on the post infusion studies. There is evidence that the mass lesion involves the habenular commissure. There is associated shift of the posterior portion of the third ventricle to the right and there is associated ventricular dilation involving the lateral ventricles, temporal horns, and the third ventricle. The pineal gland is identified.

Summary: Enhancing mass lesion anterior to the pineal primarily involving the region of the central median nucleus of the thalamus on the left but involving the habenular commissure. The nature of this lesion is uncertain. Glioma should be considered the most likely cause. Ectopic pinealoma may occur in this area but is considered rare.

We are taken to Dr. B's office
I sit down in front of her desk
Mom is sitting next to me

I have never been in a doctor's office before
having thought
examining room was the office

Dr. B looks directly at me
in a soft but firm voice
she says

what we have is a brain tumor
we have is a brain tumor
have is a brain tumor
is a brain tumor
a brain tumor
brain tumor
tumor
umor
mor
or
r.....
...
..
.

surprise
dread
numbness

we look at the scans
cloudy
foreboding ugly misalignment
they don't make sense to me
they are frightening

perhaps knowing
that I am only swallowing
bits and pieces

Dr. B speaks slowly
articulating
what is wrong
laying out a treatment plan

medication
to reduce cerebrospinal fluid inundation

hospitalization
something called an angiogram
one percent chance of having a stroke

transfer to main hospital in Los Angeles
for something called a shunt
a tube into my brain
start radiation

I'm only Seventeen and
Seventeen doesn't understand much
he wants this thing out of here
as soon as possible

he imagines
radiation might work
might get some of it
might not work at all

asks
why can't you just remove it surgically

it's much too deep
says Dr. B

much too deep
that doesn't sound good
Seventeen falls a little farther into this pit

she says
I'm going to talk with your Mom for a few minutes

Seventeen sits alone in her office
his mind is blank
shock and lethargy is buffering some of this

he and his mother walk to the car
he says
there goes Washington

she says
when this is over
you'll go to Washington

Seventeen
the newborn baby
does not have a clue
what his mother
is thinking
feeling

she says
doctor thinks this is a tumor teen-agers get
can be treated with radiation
six difficult months
and then everything should be OK

sounds acceptable
but he is still terrified

putting in a box
his hair
his head
his brain

confusing thoughts of radiation
soon to be zapped mind

a political friend will say
he doesn't know if he could have radiation

well
thanks for your perspective
fuck you

meanwhile
his third ventricle continues taking on water

he swallows pills
he barfs
he sleeps

swallows pills
barfs
sleeps

swallows pills
barfs
violently into the wastebasket next to his bed

Dr. B has given Seventeen a hopeful prognosis
but as he wretches in the dark
he wonders
is this how my life will play itself out

a few decades ago
hydrocephalus would advance unabated
his brain would squash itself

David Orenstein
1962 - 1979

now we have steroids to reduce inflammation
and relieve his third ventricle

he swallows more pills
he barfs again

his pharmacist father says
if you can keep them down
you'll feel a lot better

ads purveying mind control are recalled
playing hypnosis with friends
pop culture citations of
the power of the mind

he commits to reprogramming his brain
with a command to cease the vomiting
composing a mantra

they must stay down
they will stay down

he really is concerned
that if he's unable to digest the pills
he is in big trouble

so
he swallows pills
and repeats to himself

they must stay down
they will stay down

they must stay down
they will stay down

they must stay down
they will stay down

some time passes
without puking

they must stay down
they will stay down

allowing himself to think
this might be working
the pain starts to subside

they must stay down
they will stay down

the shroud of lethargy begins to lift

they must stay down
they will stay down

Dad asks
how are you doing

Seventeen says
starting to feel a little better

Dad says
maybe there is some hope for my profession

soon Seventeen is standing in the kitchen
eating crackers
floodwaters receding
the pain disappears
his vision re-fuses

despite his concerns
he would not have drowned
Mom or Dad would have taken him to the hospital
the steroids would have been injected

but he has won his first battle
gained a measure of control

now the reality
he has a lesion in the middle of his brain

DREAMING AN IMMACULATE CRANIOTOMY

Mom, Dad and Seventeen
sit quietly with Dr. G
in his small office

there are several books
one titled Brain Tumors
and a plastic brain
with removable parts

taking the puzzle apart
Dr. G says

there is a new surgical route
by which to attempt
extracting the lesion

his stature is beginning its ascent
Dad will call him
the Great Doctor
a play on his name

the terrified mother will say
what a man

Seventeen broods
what am I doing here

Dr. G outlines the proposed
journey through Seventeen's head

a microscope will assist
in navigating between the occipital lobes
over the cerebellum
into the midbrain
and plucking out the little troublemaker

his parents listen
while the Brain in question
tries to create an acceptable reality

it asks
what are the risks

you could lose your peripheral vision

Dad says
perhaps in part to himself
you can handle that

bargaining Brain asks
why not a shorter route

surgeon says
that is where math lives
we don't touch that

Brain whispers
there's nothing there anyway
and is glad it can still smile

on this unimaginable stage
Seventeen plots a tolerable path
through looming benevolent mutilation

Dr. G will nimbly
pluck the tumor out
from a small inconspicuous portal
cleanly and forever shut

Seventeen's shaved curls will re-sprout
he will live happily ever after
and forget the whole thing

but all Brains agree
we abhor being touched shoved and cut
having our armor pierced

Dr. G carefully asks
what do you think

Seventeen and his Brain shrug their shoulders
you are the expert they say

we'll take your parachute
and jump with you

NEUROLOGY 101

is how Seventeen's mother described her experience
as she met with Dr. G
took in medical terminology
tried to absorb it
while making it digestible for young son

yanked out of twelfth grade
he too was learning
the subject
in this new campus

high school was presenting
ten words a week
to learn and incorporate

but rarely put to use
in one ear
out the other

one lonely word
garish
turned into a nickname for a friend

the educators
much of the time
failed to capture their students' imaginations

and often
failed to command respect

Seventeen rebelled against the educational malaise
by bringing copies of
MAD Magazine
to pass time
trapped at his desk

now he is in a new classroom
with an instructor
to be revered
his language to be understood
the Great Doctor

not having to use a dictionary
learning new words
by living them

A is for Angiogram

B Biopsy

C Craniotomy

D Diplopia

E Edema

F Foley Catheter

G Germinoma

H Hydrocephalus

I Intra-Cranial Pressure

J Journal of American Neurosurgery

K Klonopin

L Lesion

M Migraine Syncope

N Neoplasm

O Occipital Lobe

P Pineal Gland

Q Quagmire

R Radiotherapy

S Scotoma

T Tomography

U Upward Gaze Paralysis and Parinaud Syndrome

V Ventriculoperitoneal Shunt

W Wallerian Degeneration

X Xanax

Y Youth

Z Zen mindfulness

not words for the SAT
not words to impress others
not words to enrich schoolboy communication
but words
to speak the language
of this nightmare

AMBULANCE TO ADULTHOOD

Arriving in the pediatric ward
Seventeen shares a small room with three other boys

two little kids
their toys balloons and stuffed animals

another about eleven
in traction
his leg in a large cast

Seventeen is the old man

steroids rendering him asymptomatic
his brain modifies a song currently on the radio
about getting out of this place

the nurse informs him
you're going to have an angiogram

I need to shave off
your pubic hair

ugh
but she says

you can do it yourself
and spare the embarrassment

Seventeen chooses to spare the embarrassment
and have some control

his pubes still a prized novelty
forty months he reckons

he survives the test without them
and the one percent chance of having a stroke

the nurses here call him David
David is now to be transferred by ambulance

from this pediatric ward in Panorama City
to neurosurgery in Los Angeles

still considering himself an able-bodied teenager
why can't he walk to the car and have Mom drive him there

he's a hospital patient
starting to feel like a basket case

so onto a gurney
wheeled to the ambulance

Mom joins him inside
she has a serious look on her face

strapped in flat on his back
one ritual after another

it continues to set in
this is a fucking serious illness

they arrive at Seventeen's new home
a hotel for adults with brain diseases

the nurses call him Mr. Orenstein
Mr. Orenstein shares a room with a grandfatherly man

the room is comfortable
three meals and his own TV

his gray-haired companion
talks about his grandchildren

Mr. Orenstein wants to be David again
he wants to be goofing off with his friends

DECEMBER 19, 1979

Days of waiting
days of lounging
days of visitors, phone calls, cards and letters
days of Mom bringing Seventeen candy and hamburgers
to the hospital
come to an end

this last day
Seventeen washes and shakes out his curls
even though they only have a few hours left

the steroids have reduced intracranial pressure
feeling fine he fancies

why can't I just keep taking these pills for the rest of my life

Mom and Dad stay through the evening
and wish him well

they appear to be calm and cheerful
Seventeen is unable
to grasp their terror

told to stop eating at midnight
he munches on brownies
and watches reruns
of Hogan's Heroes and Twilight Zone

the munching is halted at exactly 12 am
TV turned off
with little anxiety or fear
he drifts off to sleep

first glow of dawn
there is no more delay
this is it
we have to face the music

orderlies appear as scheduled
at 6:00 am
he stands up
climbs aboard the gurney
on his own

rolled down halls
through elevator doors
relishing each moment of the ride
each delay in reaching the destination
with his skull still intact

arriving in pre-op
ouch, a needle in the butt
this is Demerol they say
it will help you relax
but he is relaxed

in a few minutes euphoria
his first opioid
this is great!
he says to himself

a woman with a German accent cuts his hair
she will put the curls in a bag
what will he do with them

the hostages are being held in Tehran
and German woman says
I was in Dresden during the war
we should do that to Iran

Seventeen's curls falling away
a tumor in his brain
about to have his head cut open

he looks at the clock
7:30 am
on a normal Wednesday
Jeff's Mom would be driving the boys to school

wheeled to the operating room
bright lights
busy people in blue gowns
a table filled with scores of perfectly arranged
shiny tools and blades

Dr. G appears
from behind his mask he asks

are you ready Dave

this man
Seventeen's doctor
Seventeen's savior
Seventeen's hope
Seventeen hands himself over to him

the anesthesiologist places a hissing device under his nose
she says
count backwards from one hundred

one hundred
ninety-nine
ninety-eight
ninety-seven
ninety- six
ninety-five
ninety...

At this point, after having wrapped the legs and inserted a Foley catheter, the patient was placed in a semi-sitting position and the head secured in place with the Mayfield pin head clamp. The head was positioned directly in line with the body. The remainder of the skull was shaved. The head was then prepared in the usual fashion. Prior to final draping, landmarks were noted on the scalp and a scalp incision was then outlined using a sterile marking pen. Scalp incision started just below the inion and was carried up toward the lambda approximately 7.5cm and then miter-shaped flap was designed by dropping the lateral limb down to the asterion. The line of incision was injected with a solution of ¼% Xylocaine with epinepherine 1 : 400,000. Scalp incision was carried down to the pericranium and Raney clips were placed on the scalp for hemostasis. Scalp flap was then secured out of the immediate field of operation. The pericranium was incised with a cutting diathermy after which the inion lambda, saggital suture and asterion were all identified. A bur hole was placed just laterally and above the inion, this being just inside the junction of the superior sagittal and transverse sinuses. Another bur hole was placed directly above this, approximately 6cm toward the lambda, just off the midline. The other bur hole was placed just above and medial to the asterion. The dura was swept away from the inner skull, clearing the sagittal and transverse sinuses. Craniotome was then used to connect these bur holes, creating a free bone flap. At this point, sagittal and transverse sinuses were identified. There was good bony exposure over the transverse sinus. The dura was opened, starting at a point at the upper medial corner of the bone flap, extending to the inferior lateral corner. This was then tied to the medial inferior corner. Sutures were used to retract the dura out of the field of operation. The occipital lobe was identified and retractor was placed within the wound, retracting the occipital lobe laterally and superiorly providing exposure of the free edge of the tentorium. After covering the occipital lobe with Biocol, a Greenburg retractor was used to secure retraction of the occipital lobe off the posterior floor exposing falx cerebri and the tentorium. Silver clips were placed across the free edge of the tentorium. Groove director was used in a fashion slowly advancing as the tentorium was incised. Retraction sutures were then placed at the free edges of the tentorium this structure out of the field of operation. At this point, the operating microscope was introduced into the field. Under 10x magnification, the arachnoid over the superior cerebellar surface was identified and opened. This arachnoid was rather thick and milkish white in color. After freeing the arachnoid in the direction of the vein of Galen, the vermis then fell away from the immediate field of operation, giving good exposure of the free edge of the tentorium on the opposite side. Careful, blunt, and sharp dissection was carried out further.

Freeing the arachnoid from the complex of veins in this area. Those being the basal vein of Rosenthal and the vein of Galen and the internal cerebral veins. Further adjustment of the retractor provided a good exposure medially, anteriorly and superiorly to the venous complex, exposing the corpus callosum. In spite of various attempts at maneuvers, the pineal was not visualized. The splenium of the corpus callosum was split in the midline at a point which would be directly above the pineal gland. Upon extending the cerebrotomy anteriorly, the velum interpositum was opened, exposing the choroid plexus of the third ventricle as well as a number of large turgid arteries. After further exploration in this area, no tumor or pineal was identified. Having carried out a rather tedious dissection to this point and not having been able to identify the tumor, it was felt that further attempt to locate the tumor would present undue risks to the patient. Therefore, it was agreed upon by all neurosurgeons present that no further exploration should be attempted. After securing all small points of bleeding with the bipolar cautery, the self retaining retractors were removed. After waiting for approximately 5 to 8 minutes to further observe the area for bleeding, none was noted. The area was irrigated with Ringer's lactate solution with Bacitracin, after which the dura was closed with interrupted sutures of #4-0 black silk. Dural tenting sutures were placed along the bone margin. The bone flap was then replaced and secured into position with #28 gage stainless steel wire. Pericranium was reapproximated on all sides of the craniotomy after which the wound was closed in a two layer fashion, using #2-0 Polydek in the galeal layers, the skin being closed with #4-0 Polydek. A small Davol drain was placed in the subgaleal space and brought out through a separate stab wound. The needle, cottonoid and sponge count were correct at the end of the procedure. Estimated blood loss was 225 cc with none being replaced during the intraoperative period. It should be noted that prior to starting the bone work, the patient had received 60 mg of Lasix and 275mg of 20% Mannitol. Also, a total of 70 cc of ventricular fluid was drained by way of the external ventriculostomy. Though *not noted above, it should be pointed out that the brain was very relaxed at all times during the surgery, and at the end of the surgery, there was considerable space between cortex of the brain and the inner table of the skull overlying the right hemisphere. The patient's head was removed from the Mayfield pin head clamp, after which dry sterile dressing was applied to the wound. The ventriculostomy was connected to high pressure tubing for subsequent monitoring and interventricular pressure. The patient was transferred from the operating room to the recovery room with the endotracheal tube in place. At the time the patient left the operating room, he was not yet awake.*

after ten hours
From out of the fog
comes a voice

David, do you know where you are?

the words
Kaiser – Sunset – Hospital
emerge from bandaged exhaustion

followed by a stream of vomit
last night's brownies?
for which Seventeen meekly apologizes

unfamiliar voices acknowledge amongst themselves
that he is aware
and pardon him
for having made an unpleasant mess

in this bright florescent room
busy with activity and voices
Seventeen is drowsily half conscious
of how utterly awful and helpless he feels

devoid of energy and strength
his head is now
a turban of bandages
sutures pain and fear
he is terribly thirsty
allowed to suck on a wet cloth

feels the constant urge to urinate
and is told
that is taken care of

he becomes aware of the presence of Mom and Dad
they ask

David, how are you feeling

ok

after some hours or days
he looks around and sees blurry figures

gazes at one
is it a man
looks like one

with a beard
he thinks so

but why is it so hard for him to tell
panic ensues
what is wrong with me

Mom!

I can't see!
I'm afraid...

Seventeen was not thinking about his parents
the specter of vision loss was not only his terror

his mother faints and drops to the floor
he is later told

Dr. G assures him
the hyper-dilated pupils would accommodate
the vision would clear up

Seventeen is too scared to believe him
the doctor tests his peripheral vision
how many fingers am I holding up?

Seventeen can't see any fingers
and resigns himself to
oh well, that's gone

bargaining with a God
he never paid much attention to

ok, I'll accept this loss
if I can still
drive
read
take photographs

all without peripheral vision

the hours and days pass
lying in discomfort
while agonizing over his inability to see

there remains the larger issue
why hasn't Dr. G
a smile on his face
presented a vial containing the apprehended lesion

where is Seventeen's victory parade
the reward for this trial
when can he stop agonizing

malignant or benign
invasive or encapsulated
completely or partially resected
life or death

if death will he die
quickly and painlessly
or
a slobbering invalid

a few weeks ago Seventeen was fixated on girls
and worrying about which college to apply to

what does malignant mean anyway
at Seventeen

a capacity for empathy
is growing

lying in bed he wishes this on no one
wouldn't wish it on Hitler

Hitler!
what the fuck are you talking about!

I was really feeling bad... that's what I was thinking at the time

Hitler? that makes our story sound stupid. Hitler...

shut up, you don't remember what it was like

fuck you I don't

no, fuck you

TEN DAYS

Picture yourself
Seventeen
in the hospital intensive care unit

flat on your back
enveloped in a numbing
transcendent terror

feeling
absolutely miserable

your vision is blurry
you are exhausted
frightened and apprehensive

aware of being
utterly helpless

here and there
sensations emanating
from your bodymind

confined to an antiseptic
medical techno environment

devoid of nature
bathed in fluorescent light
without sun moon or stars

family, friends pets plants trees
bugs and spiders
supplanted by the sick and their attendants

Seventeen
you are
absolutely dependent on
nurses, doctors
and technology

to sustain and heal
this infantilized new edition of yourself

when I call to enquire about you
they say
fair condition

your legs wrapped in ACE bandages
preventing blood clots

catheter in your penis
busy draining urine
yet inducing a false and constant
urge to urinate

intravenous needles
invade the arteries of your hands and wrists

supplying fluids medications nourishment
constricting your ability to move
and as the days pass
ache and sting

pulling off the heart monitor on your chest
a faster way of getting nurses' attention

your head is wrapped in bandages
covering more than thirty sutures

three wire clips
holding together
the new trap door in your skull

a shunt tube
ascending from deep in your brain
through skull and bandages

preventing your ventricles
from wreaking intracranial havoc

the intracranial fluid rolling on
to a monitor with red LED digits

a curiosity to gaze at
while fending off your boredom and anxiety

the days have lost their names
mornings afternoons evenings
nighttime daytime

morph into a muddle
of slothfully passing time

you are vaguely aware of sharing an intimacy
with companions you will never know

a comatose adolescent motorcycle catastrophe
his parents bring Crosby Stills and Nash tunes
hoping to awaken him

wooden ships on the water soothe you
will the boy ever hear music again

a terrified aging woman beside you
panicking that she is done for
if a bowel movement doesn't come soon

you listen quietly to her desperation
you listen to her prayers

she pulls aside the curtain dividing you
exposing herself and beseeching you

Boy, see if I am going!

and from your bed you will witness
the trauma and agony
of that alcoholic's death

on Christmas day
the nurse will ask
what do you want

a younger version of yourself
now an affectation
states that he would like a car
a Corvette

but your sadness overcomes you
you tell the nurse

I just want to go home

you have found the intensive care unit
an uncomfortable frightening place
the purpose of which is
your recovery and well being

nurse brings you bed pans
wipes you clean
embarrassing

nurse gives you sponge baths
a pleasure

the strangers in this room
shepherding you from an invalid on a gurney
back to a functioning teen-ager
enabling you to

drink from a cup
pee into a pitcher
sit for a moment in a chair
until the return to gravity
overwhelms your brain

they feed you
clear liquids
then soft foods
then solid foods

they help you
stand up
walk a few steps

use a toilet by yourself
and wipe your own butt

and after ten days
your parents are permitted
to escort you out of the hospital

a few hours to reemerge into the world
whose cogs and wheels
haven't stopped turning

THE MAN IN THE INTENSIVE CARE UNIT

You were there to mend a perforated ulcer
after overdoing it on a boat
the nurses caring for you
reminding you to attend the drinkers group

I did not pay much attention to you
too busy bargaining
asking, if I get out of this
may I still read, drive and use my camera

you seemed to be in a good mood
an occasional laugh
conversation
I am looking better you told my mother

my days were catheters tubes bandages and panic
benign or malignant
was the scar too big and ugly
would I still be me

suddenly you are vomiting
stomach acid pouring into a ruptured wound
screams of agony
nurses and doctors scrambling to save you

your internal flash flood of blood and pain
washing away my adolescent veneer
of boyish pranks, sex, a license to drive

so what if I had the balls to take that Bentley
for a joyride through Benedict Canyon

the nurses tell Mom she has to leave
I have already reverted to childhood
sobbing, Mommy don't go

as your agony subsides into delirium
you beg God
I have been a good man, please

awakened by a nurse in the morning
alcohol I did not drink burning my innards
I ask about you

oh, he died last night
isn't that a shame

I am not familiar with death
that will take another couple of decades
but I am hurting inside

I tell myself
no need to feel bad about your death
you did it to yourself

the pain dissipates
and the world saw fit that I return to school
and get on with it

you lived a long life
and all I know of it
is that you bled to death beside me
I don't even know your name

HOMECOMING

Three weeks in the hospital
ten days in the intensive care unit
ten hours in the operating room
one lesion in the brain
one death of a fellow patient

up on his feet again
newly minted Seventeen
is granted a siesta

coming home to welcome the new year
new decade
new realities

wheeled to the infirmary exit
Dad helps his wobbling son to the car

amidst the traffic
it is apparent that if he ever drives again
this once second nature pleasure

now demands adjustment to
vision changes
and the specter of fear

driving
and other tasks
will now require intense concentration

beware of ghost images
scan the adjacent fields of that empty spot
take Jim Morrison seriously

keeping
his now wayward eyes
on the road

arriving
Seventeen is overwhelmed
astonished
to find his family's suburban home
transformed in his absence
to a lavish ornate museum

hardwood floor
rugs and carpeting
incandescent light
sofas, cushy chairs and coffee tables
shelves brimming with books albums periodicals
verdant house plants
Tobiasse and others adorning the walls
the Amana side-by-side full of delightful food

a mother
a father
a sister

a brother
paradise

his mental fuel tank is low
but terror has subsided
for the moment
euphoric to be standing in the kitchen

as Dorothy said
there's no place like home
no place like home

well wishers
concerned friends and relatives
keep the phone ringing

but what will he say
what does he tell them
how does one explain…

Aunt Red calls
it's good to be home
he tells her sincerely
it's good to be home

his family sits in chairs
around a mouthwatering display of ordinary food

for the first time in his presence
Dad drinks himself to tipsiness

Seventeen's Decadron hyper appetite
amusing the family
and creating explosive pain
behind his sternum

is he having a heart attack to boot
those far off adult maladies
now just around the corner

but relief dawns on Seventeen
this is what those Alka-Seltzer ads portrayed

the phone rings
Mom takes a call from Susie
Seventeen is happy she's calling
but he is vehrklempt
too much water behind the dike

Mom pleads
take the phone
the girl is crying

how totally unprepared he is
to have a brain tumor

the new year arrives
the family watches the ball drop
1980 on Seventeen's head
a new year
a new decade

and with luck
legal adulthood
graduation from high school
voting in a presidential election
Reagan or Carter

he goes to bed
in his own room
free from the ward's chatter and noise
free of blood pressure monitors
stethoscopes and thermometers

but also a night of frightful dreams
fear of neighborhood bullies pulling at his hat
insurance bureaucrats holding sway over his life

and morning comes
relatives arrive for "the game"
but football is suddenly preposterous
and painful to watch

the patient feigns his former interest in sports
smiles and attempts generating small talk
all creative cylinders firing

see my smile
I'm okay
same old me

NOT

his beloved cousin arrives
Seventeen turns on the facade
the room is noisy
TV blaring
he quietly forces the fluff
out of his mouth

but the cousin doesn't hear his words
making a
"what did you say?" face

which Seventeen construes as a
"you're not making sense" face

is some intracranial malfunction
compromising his ability to communicate
does he appear to be damaged

keep it together
don't let them sense your anxiety

be a good host
don't make anyone uncomfortable
don't let them see you falter

the phone rings
a seventeen-year-old friend
the future will grant him the crown of medical doctor
but he already thinks he is
and queries

Is it benign or cancerous

cancerous?
the word has not been uttered once
at home or hospital
since Seventeen fell into this pit

what is cancer anyway
at 206 months of age
he knows this

people who get cancer die
as they did in Love Story and Brian's Song
it eats them up and kills them

Seventeen has never heard of brain cancer
therefore brain cancer must not be him

he returns to the game
and family
who was that
they ask

it was so and so
adding
he thinks I might have cancer

Seventeen stating this is an absurdity
for his guests to chuckle at

but no one laughs
instead there is silence and solemn faces

keep it together, David
keep it together

a knock at the door
sister's friends stream in

now he really has to fake it
who the fuck are these people
the gasket bursts
why are they here

he retreats
into his room
and into bed

in time Seventeen
will make friends with anxiety
but now suspects he's losing his mind

pounding heart
tight chest
dry mouth
the urge to run away

fearing
has this past month diminished his mind
has his brain been damaged
has he changed

easy does it my friend
you are the same old you

let's be easy on ourselves
we've been through a lot
we just need some time
just need some time

Seventeen calms himself
exiting his shelter
the house is quiet
the aliens have gone home
a new person has emerged

THE NIGHTMARE

Twelve thousand nights
since leaving the hospital

all those years
I remember only two related dreams
both the first night home

dream one

neighborhood girl torments
tugging at my protective hat
she demands
what's under that

a painful situation
I don't want other kids
to see my head

in reality
only a few stupid remarks
people are helpful
or quiet

dream two

returning to the hospital
after my short visit home
a dreamy stage presents
an antiseptic entrance
flooded by fluorescent light

there is a long table
behind it cartoonish bureaucrats
with pens and paper

egghead officers
humpty dumpties
in lab coat uniforms
beady eyes behind thick glasses
ridiculous yet powerful gatekeepers

their approval required
to gain entrance

I approach
weak needy dependent
Seventeen going on seven
going on seventy

cancer in my head
sutures still in place
I must pass this inspection

approaching the table
the eggheads mumble

zha zha shu zha zha

identifying myself
and why I am here
they respond dismissively

a zhib zhub zhib zhub zhib
zhib zhib zhib zhib zhib

growing anxious I try to explain
they shake their heads

a zhib zhib zhib zhib zhib zhib
zhub zhub zhub

now trembling
I plead

I am sick
a patient here
please let me in

a zhub zhub zhub zhub zhub
zhib zhib zhib zhub zhib

tears stream
doesn't anyone understand
Please!

zhub zhub zhub zhib zhub
no no no no no

and then
the straining dam fails
exploding with a scream
at the eggheads
and at the world

I HAVE A BRAIN TUMOR

I awaken in my quiet room
shaking in a cold sweat
the howl still echoing in my head

certain the cry
has rattled the windows
and awoken my parents and sibs

waiting for my father to burst into the room
I recognize this cry
has rattled only my mind

the house is dark and silent
my father does not arrive
and the next day
I return to the hospital

for now
the gate is open
a nightmare in this awful nightmare

for now
the eggheads let me pass

BACK TO SCHOOL

This brain tumor
and its treatment
thankfully far from the frontal lobe
involved the pineal region
third ventricle, sixth nerve and occipital lobe

pressure and hydrocephalus
under control
the mind's highways operational

all factors
sparing most of Seventeen's
cognitive and other abilities

that allowed
after a nearly two-month absence
returning to school

an unnerving prospect
for an adolescent
and his vanity

pale
fatigued
nervous

wearing a beanie
to cover the wounds of thirty-six sutures
forming a large U-shaped scar
on the back of his shaved scalp

radiation targets
drawn in black ink
on each side of his head

he is not one of the popular kids
tormented those lower on the totem pole

how will they treat him
will they laugh
make comments
toy with his hat

he nervously recalls
that boy in junior high

having had brain surgery
his head shaved
he wore a wig
which was pulled off
and thrown on the floor

Ha Ha Ha

that was junior high
twelve to fourteen-year-old boys

Seventeen is hoping the fifteen to seventeen-year-olds
have grown up a bit

the school is good about accommodating him
psychologist and tutor provided
he has much missed work to complete

his teachers have been informed
ready for his arrival

he chooses the pace
one class the first week
all four after that

a few weeks ago
he was in the intensive care unit
with a Foley catheter

Mom drops him off
this is his school
he knows his way around
amidst the noise and chatter

everything is the same
but different

he meets an old friend
yeah, I heard
he says
makes a crack
and sits next to Seventeen in class

Mr. Smith
kind and understanding
he fought during the War
maybe he knows something about wounds

it's a government class
Seventeen writes weekly current events papers
the hostages in Iran

then out for another two weeks
another operation
a seizure
and back to school again

while Mom drives Jeff and Seventeen home
he has a migraine syncope
amidst the scintillations he says

don't worry Jeff
I'll be OK

his fear of scholastic torment is unfounded
most of the kids are quiet
some helpful

in photography class
they assist him with a 4" x 5" camera assignment

Mr. Carter makes a class get well portrait
and sends it to the hospital

Randy
a friend's older brother
and Scott
take him to the beach and the mountains
helping with a slide show assignment

the AP English exam approaches
over the course of the year
Seventeen has managed to read

half of Crime and Punishment
and Cliff Notes for The Jungle

he tells Ken
I am not going to take the exam
I am not prepared
not up to it

Ken encourages him
take the exam

if you get a good score
great
if you get a bad score
who cares

he takes the exam
gets a good score

and his fears of being unable to compete in college
evaporate

at the circus that was a
suburban Los Angeles high school graduation
Mark Lisa and Sue stand by him
adjust his graduation cap
make him comfortable

and with the help of his parents
family
 teachers
doctors and nurses
friends
and faith in himself

despite the last six months
Seventeen graduates high school

CRIES AND PANGS OF THE BODYMIND

In his comfortable hospital room
Seventeen's skull healing
vision improving
optimistic
loved and cared for

hope remains
they will get this thing

yet sirens and strange things emerge within him

knees aching
dizzy spells
an evening of relentless salivating

and
spirits arriving each night
upon Mom and Dad's departure
and turning off the TV

laboring in the darkness
they move slowly
purposefully
about his room

picking things up
putting things down

shadowy gray ghosts
are they there to haunt him

Seventeen decides to welcome
these visitors
and let them do their work

if they follow him home
he'll worry about his sanity

the visitors remain in the hospital
but angrier demons
grief terror trauma and rage

rioting emissaries
demanding acknowledgement
follow him home
stationing themselves throughout
his bodymind

becoming lifelong pals
squeezing poking prodding
demanding to be heard

launching muscle spasms
in his knees
back
ribs

gut
jaws
eyelids
and toes

their shock troops shuttle
through the labyrinths of his nervous system
with their migrainous arsenal

hallucinations
pain
vomiting and fainting

from where did this dark energy come

pain had been an infrequent visitor
homage to proud boyhood bruises and broken bones

his body had been
a calm and peaceful place

but Seventeen keeps on smiling
laughing
joking
clowning
intellectualizing

expecting himself
as the world expects him
to forget about it

Hey! Listen up buddy don't ignore us!

there are other changes
Seventeen immediately loses interest
in football, basketball and baseball

he avoids opening those once engrossing coffee table books
he can't hang that new Neil Young poster
he loses his interest in Porsches and P-51s
the wonder in National Geographic's accounts of planetary
    exploration
evaporates

now he finds himself
in library stacks
perusing reference books
and medical journals

brain tumors
seizures
neurosurgery
migraine
depression
anxiety
new hobbies you can't share with your friends

there are more departures from himself

Seventeen
has become easily irritated
quick to anger and picking fights

over such injustices as
discourteous driving
thoughtless comments
or nothing much at all

more dis-ease

the boy was sensitive
but Seventeen flinches
upon a warm hand on his shoulder

at the dinner table
be careful where your foot wanders
touch Seventeen's shoe
and he'll rocket through the ceiling

what is happening to him
why has he become a wound-up spring

clinicians, friends and family notice

you're a nervous kind of guy
cheer up, dude!
you're so serious
you're a hothead
we should get you a punching bag

and complete reversals

Seventeen can no longer easily imagine
a future

life has become
a perpetual fire alarm
in which to avoid disaster
keep the serpents at bay
and effect repairs

maybe
when this goal is met
he'll allow himself to hang that poster
and build a life

once upon a time
he imagined himself
a successor to Margaret Bourke-White

finding a girl
getting married
and creating a family a viable possibility

and then the future succumbed
to a singular effort to avoid falling off
this narrow bridge

who will he become

he was told
laugh and the world laughs with you
cry and you cry alone

so who will he be
a smiling inappropriate affectation
a divided self

or an authentic man
at ease
with grief and tears

WELCOME TO MIGRAINEVILLE

After two months
marble remains
in Seventeen's brain

he has become
a smiling mask
all is fine
a model of bravery and resilience

fine brave enraged
fine brave terrified
fine brave foreboding

a house of cards
a youthful assemblage
of adult terror
and unmanageable feelings

he sits comfortably
watching reruns

suddenly
a firefly

optical illusion
appears on his occipital projection screen
a strobe-light
of intensely pure
primary colors

this unrequested presentation
met by fear and anxiety

what is my fucking brain doing now

is this an alarm
a hemorrhage
intracranial pressure
wounded neurons crying out

what now

Seventeen has become skillful
calming himself
with fanciful diagnostic concoctions

this event must be
his swollen occipital lobe
shrinking
creating cartoons
as it crinkles back to normal

the show persists for several minutes
then vanishes

what the hell was that

stay calm
you've been through a lot
everything is going to be OK
your brain needs time to heal

months later
after fainting spells
the onset of pain
diagnosis will be made

Seventeen is inducted into the helotry
of migraine

a tormenting enigma
with a life of its own
storming in uninvited
unexpected
absconding on holiday

mild
violently aggressive

he will appear
again
again
and again

while hanging with friends
in the hospital parking lot
on Yom Kippur
preparing dinner for a girl
visiting the grandfather of a friend

while swimming
driving on the Ventura freeway
at an Italian eatery with family
in front of the computer at work
in the middle of a dream

vision invaded by strobe lights
expanding checkerboards
scintillating doughnuts
lines pops squiggles
flak and shrapnel

often followed by
throbbing pain
and profound sense
of non-well-being

during the first raps at your door
you can drive through blind spots
perhaps over the boy
running into the street

you can speak
through disconnected voice

you can walk
into a door

pain arrives
throbbing gritty nauseating
pain

he goes where he wants
from place to place
within the upper right quadrant of the head
hopping skipping surfing
visiting the left side
sinus caverns
neck
the hole drilled for a long obsolete shunt

pulsating
throbbing

you crave darkness
light is tortuous

you crave quiet
sound is noise

conversation
while possible
heavy and excruciating
for spitting out facts and requests

incoming words
if not soft empathetic
are blackboard fingernails

intuition says
curl up in a warm bed
hide in a dark room
sounds comfortable

you never get there
he is after you
you can't lie still

you sit
you walk
you moan
you toss and turn
you cry out

you think pain
live for its cessation

he plays this game for hours
days for some

he laughs at your snake oils
and pokes
you paid for this

he hides behind narcotics
waiting to return

in the emergency room
they injected opioids

Seventeen went home
migraine was in the back seat
waiting

willpower allows masquerading
for a time
but you are overcome

Seventeen made many pilgrimages
clutching the crapper
barfing until his stomach was spent
then dry heaving
as if to extricate

the lesion
the hospital
the dying patients
terror and grief
his scarred head
torn dura
aborted childhood
rage at nature
or God

and then
the pain subsides
cleansed and euphoric
he gets up
gets something to eat
and starts all over again

TONIC - CLONIC

Trying to present as
acclimated
strong
resilient
pushing himself through

another operation
inserting a tube to drain fluid
like swatting a flea
compared to December 19

Seventeen awakens
how easy this is now

several days to recuperate
no sweat

he likes the hospital food
likes the attention

dinner in bed
a friend calls
not coming to visit
he met a girl

disappointed
Seventeen returns to his fried chicken
and chocolate pudding
yum

a new lease and loathe on life
foreign valves and hoses
will let him go to school
and hang with friends

in these roller coaster months
there is belief that he will get out of this
acceptably scathed
and rejoin the world

he is enjoying his chocolate dessert
Suddenly

darkness

- - - - - - - - - -

he emerges
disoriented
splattered with pudding

where am I
what room is this
why am I weak
wrapped in bandages
food in my face

his father says

David

you are in the hospital
you had a s_____

oh no

whimpering
as reality rushes in

the absence
momentarily hiding
brain tumor

dread awareness
this is a game changer

control
disability
girls
school
cars
career
manhood
normalcy

who is going to love him

how can he keep mending
this tearing fabric

on call doctor appears
not Dr. G
who would show concern
and help Seventeen absorb

Dr. Strangeperson says
yup, a s_____
yup, the hard drive crashed
yup, the car is totaled

Seventeen asks
will it happen again

probably

as if he has asked an annoying question

the response
breaks his thin ice
he plunges into a freeze

the remaining week in the hospital
can barely speak
barely eat
walks in a slow shuffle
vision worsens

Mom says
they can be controlled
she is right
but the unspeakable words

s e I z u r e

e p I l e p s y

hang over him
he cannot vocalize this new reality

when Susie visits a month later
he will invent an acceptable term

he had
a black out

he returns home deflated
but able to walk talk and eat
trying to start the healing again

into his warm bed
and God laughs

he is met by a new
excruciating pain
a bee sting
scorpion bite
or gunshot

retreating into the fetal position
the pain is not in his head
or at the surgery sites

this pain
searing from the embarkation point
of a once assumed future family
screaming

WHAT IS HAPPENING TO ME

MERRITT AND PUTNAM'S DILANTIN ISLAND

Surmounting the breakers that imprisoned him
Tom Hanks pauses amidst triumph
gazing at the island raft that sustained his life

such an island has been a friend to Seventeen
an orange and white capsule
Phenytoin sodium 100mg aka Dilantin

having been conscripted to the tonic - clonic club
Seventeen agonizes over the specter of epilepsy
and its convulsive cocktail

shock
embarrassment
terror
dread
foreboding
hyper self-consciousness
lashed to the loss of consciousness

if he survives the lesion
what life is there to live
eyes rolling back
spasms

public vomiting
and incontinence

frightening scenes in the town square
anytime anywhere

but Mom encourages Seventeen
though he is skeptical
the attacks can be controlled

and his stormy brain
is loaded with medicine's first miracle
for calming intracranial typhoons

phenobarbital is a blessing
and a curse

freeing him from seizures
while descending into schlepping lethargy

if he survives the tumor
the convulsions halted

how will he engage in the world
alertness and energy
memories of childhood

it is however
the best of times to face seizure disorder

in thousands of generations of convulsive disease
Seventeen has the good fortune

to land in the world
with Tracy J. Putnam and H. Houston Merritt

you've never heard of Merritt or Putnam
have you

Seventeen's heroes were rock
stars and professional athletes

and they will be until he appreciates
the sparing of millions
from seizure disorder

amidst 1938's darkness
Putnam and Merritt create Dilantin

enabling some of us
to sit in classrooms
drive cars
go out on dates
stand at a podium and speak
walk on the beach
fly
without fear of seizures

Dilantin is not perfect
it can't help everyone
but thank god for Putnam and Meritt

hey Dilantin!

COMPUTERIZED AXIAL TOMOGRAPHY TWO

Proving inoperable
the lesion evades biopsy
they don't know what it is

benign
maybe it won't grow

an aneurism
maybe it burst and faded away

but the ventricles refill
every time we discontinue the meds

something's still in there

Name: David Orenstein
Date of Birth: May 18, 1962
Date of Exam: March 3, 1980

Report: When compared to the last examination, there has been a definite increase in size of the lateral and third ventricles. The enhancing parapineal tumor is again identified and shows the size to be slightly more prominent.

Impression: 1) Probable increased tumor mass size.
*   2) Definite increased lateral and third ventricular size.*

yes it's growing
but maybe this will play to my favor

my stealthy
but now apparently fast growing
malignant assassin

may be unable to hide from
phasers and photon torpedoes

RADIATION WILL MAKE YOU LIKE NEW

Every generation has its monsters
terrors to fear
in 1980 for Seventeen
it was nukes and radiation

thirty five years from
Nagasaki and Hiroshima
living with cold war
megatons aimed at everyone
drop drills and reactors on the blink

radiation was and is a loaded word
a dreaded word
a word that threatens the future

it shatters chromosomes
spawns mutations
burns and kills

but also disposes of cancer cells

surgery had not removed
the lesion in Seventeen's brain
and now the doctors turned to radiation

one friend said
I don't know if I could do that

but Seventeen's concerns had been
baseball, cars, and girls
he dreaded losing his hair

Dr. V is the radiologist
confidence radiating
from Indian accented voice
he proclaims

RADIATION WILL MAKE YOU LIKE NEW

five thousand six hundred rads
six weeks
three days per week

Seventeen's father says
let's fry the goddamn thing out of there

Seventeen imagines burned Japanese children
their skin hanging
American soldiers sickened at test sites
Hanford, Three Mile Island
and there will be Chernobyl and Fukushima

three times a week
Seventeen and Dad make the pleasant trip
down the Ventura and San Diego freeways
past the guy selling oranges at the off ramp

along Pico boulevard
and to the hospital

large, strong hands of
the technician
do the work
gently positioning Seventeen's surgery-healing head
into the sites of the weapon
and flipping the switch

he is soft spoken
Seventeen is scared
they are quiet

in the most direct way
the technician eliminates this terrible disease
and preserves Seventeen's life

like fire
which both incinerates and provides warmth
radiation heals and destroys

Seventeen tells himself
maybe curls will be spared
but one morning
they appear on his pillow
the beginning of a mass relocation
from scalp to pillow to trash can

his intuition whispers
they're gone forever

unlike his curls
the tumor cells, unseen and unnoticed
are being flushed down the toilet
and within months
the lesion is disposed of

once again, Seventeen and I have our life
our now radiated life

there will be a future
school, work, relationships
celebrations
cluster headaches, breakdowns, hospitalizations
and false alarms
fear and hope
time bombs and pots at the ends of rainbows

high risk, they will call me
pre-existing this and that

radiation
radiation
radiation will make you
radiation will make you
radiation will make you…

SUSIE AT THE EPICENTER OF BUDDING LOVE AND BRAIN CANCER

I meet Susie
at seventeen

a summer at
leadership training camp

attracted to her
exotic suburban DC origins
auburn hair
and freckles

the way she smiled
at my way of seeing things

and the face she made
when I was talking shit

the summer ends
letters fly

kissing the envelopes
as I drop them in the mailbox

an invitation arrives

she says
come to my prom!

yes
it's getting better all the time

and then
after unanswered calls
Mom tells her

bypassing a fear of flying
she journeys to California

where despite my recent happenings
with the help of friends

I arise to be
an adequate tour guide

Disneyland
whales and movie stars

she buys me a button that declares
Think Positive

is entertained by the doctor
at the radiation clinic

at lunch
she cheers me on
as I struggle to ingest
 a tiny sandwich

arriving after midnight
my sibs and parents asleep
we sit in my bedroom and talk

months earlier
I may have found myself thinking
In that boyish kind of way

now Susie is with me at my nadir

so rather than dance
the adolescent dance

I'm sharing my fresh and anguished insights
on the fragility of the brain

It's who you are
I stumble

trying to convey
its centrality to ourselves as our selves
and the dread I may be injured

we say our good-byes at the airport
Dad drives me home

how nice to have an attractive young woman
in my room on a dark and quiet night

giving me hope
and a reason to carry on

COMPUTERIZED AXIAL TOMOGRAPHY THREE

Six weeks and three thousand rads

Name: David Orenstein
Date of birth: May 18, 1962
Date of Exam: April 23, 1980

Comparison with the study of March 7, 1980, again identified is the ventricular shunt device. The ventricles are normal in size and have decreased compared to the study of March 7, 1980. The parapineal tumor is again identified but appears smaller in size as compared to the March 7, 1980 study. The previously identified mass effect of the tumor with slight left to right shift of the calcified pineal has decreased almost to midline.

Following the infusion of contrast, no abnormal areas of enhancement are identified. The parapineal tumor does not enhance on this study

IMPRESSION: Compared to the study of March 7, 1980, there has been further decrease in the ventricular size and decrease in the pineal tumor size.

The news appears to be good. My parents go outside and dance and scream. I am quiet and subdued. I notice my mother's tears. I feel satisfied but, at the same time, numb.

COMPUTERIZED AXIAL TOMOGRAPHY FOUR

Name: David Orenstein
Date of Birth: May 18, 1962
Date of Exam: August 13, 1980

REPORT: *the ventricular shunt device remains in place. The ventricles are normal in size similar to the examination on April 23, 1980.*

The previously described parapineal tumor is no longer identified. The third ventricle is midline and there is no detectable shift of the calcified pineal. Following infusion of contrast material, no abnormal areas of enhancement are seen; no abnormal enhancement in the parapineal area is noted.

The area of encephalomalacia involving the right occipital lobe is again noted and unchanged. Abnormal increased density in the right maxillary sinus is consistent with maxillary sinus disease.

IMPRESSION: *1) Normal sized ventricular system unchanged since April 23, 1980 with shunt in place.*
2) The previously described parapineal tumor is no longer identified.
3) Right maxillary sinus disease.

With the exception of a stuffy nose, it appears that I have a clean bill of health.

LIKE DOLPHINS

In the depths of winter
darkness and despair

comes care concern support and generosity
from family friends caretakers teachers
community

a giant pod of dolphins
a thousand little nudges
keep us afloat

yes, it takes a village
to heal a child

the villagers

keep on calling

bake everything I ask for

bring food to the house

send Captain America to the hospital

send gourmet popcorn to the ICU

send a plant
that lives with me in the hospital
and comes home alive

send Weegee's photos to the hospital

complete my collection of Beatles' albums

send movie passes

share a tooth brush

make a class get well photo

watch over my little brother

comfort my mother and father

offer financial help

pray for me

call the hospital operator each day
D.O. fair condition

fly across the country to accompany me

say: we'll take this one day at a time

take me for walks in the hospital

take me to UCLA

offer friendship as fellow cancer patients

act as chauffeurs

help me with class assignments

step in when I'm being harassed

see that I finish my work and graduate high school

adjust the graduation cap on my complex head

watch over me when I am able to venture far from home

calm me when I panic

have faith in me and support my dreams

THIS IS HOW I SEE THE WORLD

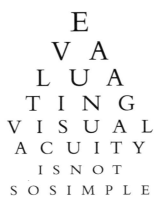

Part one

This is what happened to my Brain and Vision

nerve directing eye movement
injured by tumor

eyes no longer work together
one wanders
Brain unable to fuse their competing images
farewell to binocular vision and stereopsis

This is how I see the world

with double vision
two of everything

a world where everyone I see
has a conjoined twin

and no more life in three dimensions
no more depth perception
my world is flat

This is what happens

difficult to locate things in space
I reach for something and often miss

head miscommunicates with hands
clumsy and slow
please don't throw anything in my direction
it may bypass my uncoordinated semi-blinded hands
bounce off my fingers and hit me in the face

head miscommunicates with feet
difficult to estimate where steps are
as I descend stairways
where exactly do I place each foot

difficult to negotiate cracks and ruptures on the sidewalk
muscles and bones nervous and tense
they fear stumbling tearing fracturing

and those annoying duplicate images
must often be turned off by closing an eye
and sacrificing its useful presentations

but there is something more distressing
more frustrating

I want direct human contact
eyes to eye
or right between your eyes

but now I really do
look you eye to eye

while my other eye wanders
and your twin floats about

I sense your puzzled expression
do you appreciate your binocular vision

Part two
This is what happened to my Brain and Vision

scarring in the area of the brain that presents vision

This is how I see the world

a blind area immediately to the left of center

This is what happens

it often requires time and effort
to find the thing I want to look at

when I look straight at you
the right side of your face is missing

how often I fail to recognize
faces I know so well
when I try to read
I look at the word
shell
and see
hell

I read slowly and carefully
always looking to the left
to discover what's in that emptiness

looking at the numbers
8+1+1=10
I see
1+1=10

I balance the checkbook slowly and carefully
get frustrated and make mistakes

always looking
up and down
back and forth
so as not to miss any numbers
or oncoming cars
hiding in that hole

Part three
This is what happened to my Brain and Vision

fluid leaking in my right eye scarring the retina

This is how I see the world

With that eye
diminished acuity
lack of contrast
night blindness
yellow color blindness

This is what happens

can no longer read with my right eye
and additional clumsiness
down the staircase
negotiating sidewalk ruptures
walking in darkness
distinguishing pavement markings

and driving at night
no more of that

in the darkness
I drove into a yellow pole
broke my sternum
and destroyed my car

Part four
This is what happened to my Brain and Vision

migraine

This is how I see the world

through migraine aura hallucinations
strobelighting primary colors
zig zagging lines
popping bubbles
ghostly beasts and monsters
partial blindness

This is what happens

I can hardly see
frightened
incapacitated
life comes to a halt

Epilogue
This is what happened to my Brain and Vision

diplopia
scotoma
retinopathy
migraine

This is how I see the world

double vision
blind area
diminished retina
migraine auras
all dancing together

This is what happens

I slice onions while making breakfast
Brain screening both
onion as observed by right eye
and onion observed by left

they float and bobble next to each other

my hand must quickly determine
which image to target

at the same time
part of my left index finger
holding the onion
falls into blind spot

amidst this conflicting
duplicated and diminished imagery

I aim knife at onion
and slice my finger
as blood soaks onion
the zig zag lightning bolts of migraine aura
emerge from the upper left quadrant of visual field

behind the advancing geometric illusions
is blindness

I have two or three minutes
to get this bloody mess in order
retreat into bed

and hope this will not evolve
into six hours of agonizing pain

I want quiet and darkness
and pray that my vision will not be called upon
to read a first aid manual
or drive someone to the hospital

can you understand
that vision is often not seamless
the world is not the world you think you see

but rather the creation of a production crew
inside your head
who all show up to work each day

AUDITORY ISOLATION: THIS IS HOW I HEAR THE WORLD

Remember that childhood debate
would you rather be deaf or blind

Helen Keller said

Blindness cuts us off from things,
deafness cuts us off from people.

I emerge with visual challenges
but the nightmare has also damaged hearing

on the phone
soon after radiation

I find myself favoring my left ear
the right having lost some ability

within months
I will become
quite sensitive to noise

hyperacusis
a new

ever intensifying
lifelong companion

I begin taking flight from clamorous gatherings
or don't go at all

when venturing into the world
I stuff my ears with plugs

at thirty-four
often pleading
say that again

around forty
tinnitus

roaring hissing and ringing
has become frequent
and often loud

at forty-eight
auditory calamity

I awaken
my right ear screaming
mauled by sensorineural hearing loss

when this happens
The doc says
we throw everything at it

steroids are thrown
without success

but exacerbate
the latecomer visual ailment
central serous retinopathy

and within my trusty
dominant right eye
rods and cones inundated

yellow replaced by mud
contrast and clarity diminished

no more reading
for you my ocular pal
our wandering weakling
to the left
now has your job

and no more driving at night
in rain
with less than
optimal conditions

my Civic
now in the junkyard

this bi-sensory episode
concluding with dead and injured cilia
in my right cochlea

I am now
as they say
deaf in one ear

and in one day
the world shifts
from stereo to mono

voices fade further away
mechanisms necessary
for pinpointing the location
and range of your voice
disabled

withdrawal and loneliness

would you rather be partially blind or partially deaf

some of you have made
painful gaffs

of visual clumsiness
and confusion

but auditory deficiencies
really set you off

oh to see the wincing faces
of unstrung friends and family
upon confronting our auditory troubles

shock
impatience
perturbation

some are empathetic
patient and helpful

some laugh
roll their eyes
make clumsy jokes

exhibiting their frustration
and ignoring ours

a boss pounds his desk
when I can't hear his instructions

the Torah says
Thou Shalt Not Curse The Deaf

I need so much
to hear what you are saying
yet after that second or third appeal

what

you roll your eyes
turn your heads
and say

oh forget it!

it's not just that
you need to raise your voice

yes I am partially hearing
yet rattled
by ambient noise

entombed
in restaurant chatter

deafened
by road racket
rock and roll
TV and radio
leaf blowers and vacuum cleaners
Harleys and screaming kids

add to this
the sirens
hissing broken pipes
and discordant babble
in the loneliness of tinnitusville

life becomes a
painful cacophony

discussion
conversation
communication

crippled

and I am sorry
my hearing aid often doesn't help
ear trumpets and cupped hands far superior

reading lips
is not as easy as it may seem

and sign language
well, will you learn it too

such is partial deafness

I am thankful
very thankful
that I can still offer you one functioning ear

in a silent meadow
desert
park
or quiet room with good acoustics

life is
communicating
with people
I want so much to hear
what you are saying

MULTITASKING

Eighteen months after radiation
John and Seventeen on their way to school

engaged in lively discussion
the Clash, the Ayatollah or the girl just met

as Seventeen drives and fires off opinions
John shouts

what the fuck are you doing

Seventeen responds

what

friend says

you're driving fifteen miles per hour
in a forty-five mile per hour zone!

Seventeen smiles

shuts up
speeds up

aware that within his brain
the mental task of engaging in discussion

severely impaired
his ability to drive a car

but just two years ago he was quite
the skilled reckless driver

at ease at ninety-five
in forty mile per hour zone

yapping with friends
while racing another delinquent

his eyes on the road
on the lookout for cops

determined to defeat his opponent
in this foolish contest

yes he should have been arrested
yes he should have had his license suspended

but what happened to his ability
to be a multitasking delinquent

MEMORIES OF MEMORY

Seventeen lives on first floor
neighbor he worries about
lives on second floor

he puts egg in saucepan
lights up stove

he goes to next room
surfing the web
he hears

BOOM

oh no
did neighbor
blow her brains out

he runs outdoors
runs up stairs
pounds on her door

neighbor opens door
she says

what

Seventeen returns to his apartment
walks into kitchen

white and yellow speckles
now adorning walls and ceiling
egg and water no longer in saucepan

those five thousand six hundred rads
of field radiation

that melted the tumor away
and saved his life

may have taken a ransom
of short-term memory

and so Seventeen came into the world
losing keys
forgetting pills taken

closing the door to the medicine cabinet
and with it the knowledge that he just brushed his teeth

he will roam parking lots
fretting his car was stolen

and suffer that accusation
from the frustrated
and their forgotten words

YOU DON'T LISTEN TO ME

THE HOT HEAD

Into adulthood
temper tantrums appear

upsetting Seventeen's young brother
who once idolized the prankster

now burned by the anger
brother calls him

Hot Head

Seventeen the hot head explodes in parking lots
on the freeway
in the clinic upon bad news
at work confronting
other blistered spirits

he has become
a smiling short fuse

while driving
he mistakenly obstructs a crosswalk
the path of an older man

who slaps the car
in frustration

tripping Seventeen's alarm
sending him off to war

stampeding from the Honda
to challenge the gray-haired assailant

Seventeen adds to the display
a large rock

a woman shouts
you leave him alone

past twenty-five
Seventeen has a pre-frontal cortex
it shrieks

WHAT ARE YOU DOING

Hot Head slithers back into his hole
Seventeen says

we have a problem

aware of the rage
but at who or what
the environment that may have poisoned
the god not acknowledged
a gene evolved to manufacture tumors

Mom suggests a punching bag
brother calls him Hot Head
girlfriend sees passion
friends turn away from bitterness

one recoiling from an outburst
responds like a guru

David, you must learn to control your anger!

he tells a psychologist
give me a baseball bat
I want to smash everything to pieces

but he is alive
given a second chance
there is sublimation
yet the beast still finds exits

migraine
breakdowns
tantrums
pain and spasms
running away
refusal to embrace life

he wonders if CSN sang
no choice but to carry on
at the performance he had to miss

he turns to therapists
turns to religion
turns to meditation

embracing empathy
compassion
forgiveness
gratitude

we keep trying
we keep trying
by honoring an elderly man's effort
to cross the street

THE UNCLE HARRY SYNDROME

Uncle Harry lived large
he came to America
and paved his streets with gold

started off hawking newspapers

EXTRA EXTRA
READ ALL ABOUT IT
BIG TRAIN WRECK ON LAKE MICHIGAN!

he drank at weddings and bar mitzvahs
grabbed the mic
singing in a raspy Yiddish voice

some rolled their eyes
the boys idolized and loved him

he was found lying on his lawn
the stroke robbing him of half his body

at thirteen Dad was driving his dozing uncle's truck
upon awakening
Harry yelled
vee gayst du!

(where are you going)

no more of that
only fond recollections
that bring sad smiles

with therapy and a walker
the doctors said
he could stroll again

instead he became a ghost
haunting the nursing home for a decade

his wife was a saint
fans visited and tried to cheer him
but he lost interest in life

the motivation
to embrace therapy and walker
dead

EXTRA EXTRA
READ ALL ABOUT IT
BIG TRAIN WRECK ON LAKE MICHIGAN!

there was no discussion in the family
about the frightening consequences
of an asphyxiated brain

therapy and walker became the mantra
sublimating dread of such fate

as Uncle Harry lost himself
amidst atrophy and depression

some said
he chose this path

the dead and wounded
of his cerebral symphony
could not cry out
we are mourning
we have drowned

EXTRA EXTRA

that brain damage is enigmatic
that he may have been
overwhelmed
grief stricken
clinically depressed

soon Seventeen would have a toe in one of his uncle's shoes
feel the tug of despair
angered each time he heard the accusation
Brain does that to itself

BIRTH OF AN EMPATH

According to Webster

Empathy: the projection of one's own personality into the
    personality of another in order to share in the other's
    emotions, thoughts, or feelings

this had not been Seventeen's previous experience

picked on occasionally
he tormented
those more awkward and vulnerable

the meek boy with poor vision
the girl with myoclonic seizures
the lonely voice reaching out for companionship

and then he got whacked

a rattled brain
loss anger and fear
sadness and grief

yet conversely
amidst that gray and white matter

grow mirror cells
and a new sense appears

he says to a friend
as one would divulge an illness

I feel other people's pain

this is what happens
his father develops enlarged prostate
Seventeen is frequently rushing to the latrine

friend is beset with acid reflux
he experiences burning in his chest

sister has abdominal surgery
he has spasms in the gut

friend endures chemo
he becomes nauseous

but these odd perceptions
often prove helpful

offering empathic sympathy
to others in distress

like that astonished pariah
who exclaimed

you understand!

no these qualities did not emerge
from reflection and practice

they sprouted like obligate seeders
after the fire

MIGRAINE: MY WORLD AND WELCOME TO IT

2 November 2012
age fifty-one

a vicious aura appears
in the form of scintillating dagger
slashing into right visual field

groggy in bed
I pick up pen and paper
might be around midnight

straining to see clock through peripheral vision
as center is blind

they're coming now every few days
Google said
try cocoa

I've felt chocolaty for twelve days
do you know the pleasure
of twelve days without migraine

but Hershey hopes dashed
like all those pills

avoiding caffeine
supplements
anger workshops
headache clinics
biofeedback
neurofeedback
and magnets

all defeated

this aura is marching to its own tune
laughing at the snake oils and their purveyors
who
quacking up the wrong trees
all want the Nobel Prize

perhaps
my graine is
dis eased spirit

saying
fuck all that shit
let me talk

meanwhile
back in bed
terror and blindness

what shall I do

I can't see what I'm writing
someone coughs in another room
I will not tell anyone what is happening

yes, cocoa felt mildly high
for twelve days
maybe just maybe
I hoped

but that dagger came roaring
I don't care how good you feel
I'm coming

twelve nice days
this dagger aura is mean
and angry

maybe this is a stroke
maybe this is the one that will kill me
or leave me totally disabled

and then
the scintillating saber starts to run out of gas
and returns to its cave

but this is not over
scintillations fade
but I'm still blind
army of pain massing

why does this mind attack itself

this aura new different
aggressive short vicious
occluding center of vision

my Brain is a migraine machine
early stage pain
presenting behind right eye
pain still weak
hoping it will retreat

and
from the emptiness
some vision appears
it is 2:35 am

partially blinded
as I write
and quite calmly terrified

the pain still ready to attack
will this be six-hour agony
or fade away

I want to turn off the light
and close my eyes
stop trying to write

want to scream for help
terror and frustration

when I'm back
I'll call Cindy McCain

the senator's wife
she knows this scourge

perhaps you can see
how this hell
generates cornball thoughts

migrained mind
jumps from here to there
no peace
I was reading Tolstoy when this started

perhaps the hormones on this pain mission
dispatched from
rudimentary regions of my soul
without words
communication via
inflammation and pain
saying

LISTEN UP ASS HOLE

STOP DISSING ME

STOP IGNORING MY FRUSTRATION

STOP PRETENDING YOU ARE BRAVE

ACKNOWLEDGE MY RAGE

FEEL MY TERROR

STOP BEING A CLOWN

WIPE AWAY THAT SMILE

but I was told
laugh and the world laughs with you
cry and you cry alone

I wear my happy face
kind and funny
I say its all OK
I say take it in stride
I say forgive and forget
I take shit
and try to make lemonade
out of lemons

one said
you had brain cancer
you should be dancing in the streets

now how the hell dance with an imploding brain
what can one say

the exhausted mind
needs to rest

2:47 am
more mild pain
and now nausea

a vicious aura

outsiders ignorant
of the terror and hell of this

Bill doesn't know me
Donny doesn't understand

I see my words
are failing

pain only minor so far
I am very tired
will try to sleep

36-hour reprieve
sleep and idle bliss

3 November 2012
10:43 AM

with relief and enthusiasm
I wake up start breakfast
and a new day

and

doughnut aura appears
scintillating checkerboards

large lower left quadrant blind areas
with vague borders

transition to pain
panic and non-well being

maybe something doesn't want me
to write memoir

maybe my brain says
what about others
just forget about it

this aura not as vicious
as my new friend last night
this is familiar

pops zigs and zags
soon transitioning
to unexplainable disruptive visual activity
partial blindness
headache

becoming mentally fatigued
need to bow out

fear and apprehension
what if this happened in a real crisis
robbery
crash
earthquake
someone else's cardiac event

how many times
have I wasted a meal

ended a conversation
fled from work
pulled the car over

another day stolen
so many wasted

11:05

intense pain behind right eye
tension in face, jaw, neck, upper back

disease
dis ease

11:18 AM

vision improving
pain increasing

hard to think and write
need to lie down
engulfed by pain

tense
nervous
fearful
frustrated
angry
disappointed
disgusted

no wonder I'm not married
who wants this

I've had enough
I try to sleep

ZZZ

LOVE IS AN OPIUM POPPY

Seventeen is twenty-four
finished college in five years
and passed that other five-year mark

happy affectations working like charms

school has been
a successful attempt to run away

keep busy
have fun
don't look back

living
yet I can't break ground
on a life
embrace a discipline
imagine

a career
marriage
family
future

but I flourish in studentville
enjoying classes
playing the field

convincing myself that real life will
magically
work itself out

I can be charming
hiding the scars
not lacking for female companionship

have morphed
from barely being able to talk to girls
to surrounding himself with them

how I need
young women

surrogate nurses doctors
therapists and lovers

I have unwillingly become
empathetic

phone ringing
a good listener
the girls love it

one will whisper
because you have a feminine side
thank my cephalic battleground for that

though at some point
in this prosperity
I always run away
from intimacy

I like girls
the plumbing works
despite the wounds
I am a reasonable facsimile
of a normal young man

or maybe not

I am to some degree
successfully orchestrating
a clever masquerade

cloaking scars and deficits
laughing off confusion and grief

auditory damage
visual impairment
exaggerated startle response
processing speed
loss of ability to multitask
catch a football
or look lovingly into the eyes of a woman

just take it in stride
bury the rage
and don't reveal

the concern of being unable to support myself
(or anyone else)
that fear of harboring deadly genes
the dread of fathering metastatic offspring

let others write the script
you are resilient
you've handled this so well
an inspiration

how I feed on opioid evaluations
fueling the alter ego playing this role

when something is forgotten or dropped
just smile or make them laugh

youth hurls one forward

II

going to a movie with Sam
I collide with a girl

engaging in easy conversation
she is attractive
smart
there are smiles and laughter
energy

she has a boyfriend
the guard says
forget about her

she wants to see a movie
I back off

Sam is watching
he's a lady's man
always has girlfriends
I trust his judgment

he whispers
get her number

I say
boyfriend

he says
forget about it
she's beaming at you

yes
she's beaming at me
we exchange numbers

four hours on the phone
the girls in the house giggling

I'm in love
I tell them
and I think I really am

we see movies
hang with friends

I write her poems
she brings me books
I make her milkshakes
perfect consistency she says

aura comes
as I make burritos for her
scintillations obscuring my view

I cut myself and bleed
attempting to gracefully open
Rosarita's temporarily invisible can

my enchanting guest
giggles good naturedly
maybe she thinks I'm nervous

we have meals
absent of migraine

gazing into her eyes
all four of them
she responds
with a perplexed smile

diplopia diplopia

I don't know
if she knows

on a moonlit
snow blanketed night

we agree to watch TV
at her place

walking together
amidst the quiet snow

the only world
our conversation and laughter

a fairy tale scene
in this wintery college town

it is quite
romantic

I really think
I might love her

we arrive
TV forgotten
in her room
standing face to face

I say
is something going to happen with us

she says
I hope not
citing the absent boyfriend

train screeches to a stop
did I delude myself

why did you bring me here

exiting in the morning
disappointed

fate continues to bring us together
alarm is ringing
I don't listen

she asks
can I stay with you for the break
maybe she's changed her mind

how can I turn down
the anodyne
that girls have become

allowing me to love myself
despite the scars

her mother calls
you should eat kale she says

we are a nice couple
kale and chocolate milk shakes

living together in my room
her pile of mail beckoning
I open Pandora's box
she's writing about us

saying
I have never gotten so close
to someone so fast
but
he is the most intensely ugly person I have ever met
if it wasn't for that...

train jumps the tracks

I don't know why those words came from her
her criteria for ugly
I am amplifying this beyond

not her type
unattractive
too close
no prospects
ugly in a normal way
too skinny
too Jewish
geek freak spaz nerd wimp loser

I've heard that all before
without crashing

but every element of my spirit says
that damaged sixth cranial nerve
wandering eye
radiation burns
various and sundry injuries and scars

have made me
an unlovable freak

my sublimations shatter
and this adolescent soap opera
casts me into the trauma pit

friends suggest
talk to her

we meet
she is open
kind
considerate
not angry that I violated her privacy

patiently
holding my hand
as I fall apart

we both know
this is over the top

spring arrives
friends console me
get me a job
suggest therapy
and Fleetwood Mac songs

at twenty-four
in collegeville

still fueled to play
this well populated field

and find women
with whom to
avoid intimacy

but we meet again
walk along the lake

why can't I let go
what hasn't healed

she brings me books
my response
panic and anxiety

I resolve to pull away
acknowledge the need for counseling

I work
socialize
and continue listening to Fleetwood Mac

in these running away years
I am not conversant with
grief
trauma
anxiety
depression

or that wimpy sissy girly word
feelings

it has been less uncool
in post-brain tumor days
to fear and address tumor relapse
rather than difficult feelings

I sound the alarm to Mom
call Dr. G

he says
doesn't sound like relapse

but these still are
brain tumor days
mixed with Fleetwood Mac

nothing like a sappy love song
which croons something like

did she provoke me to weep
cause a breakdown
and destroy my delusions of love

well not exactly
she shattered my illusions of denial
allowing me to collapse
begin to acknowledge
this problem needs to be addressed

so what am I to do
keep busy
find a psychotherapist

and

like some other kids who suffer and navigate brain tumors
take the path of
I'll show you

and run run
run to graduate school

LOVE IN A TIME OF POST TRAUMATIC STRESS

Thirty years old
twelve have passed
since the derailment
I have emerged seemingly intact
deficits still hidden in the closet

living day to day
semester to semester
year to year

my goal not to articulate a future
a career
relationship with a woman
family and children
but to elude anxiety and fear

disaster might be around the corner
who can think about marriage
raising children
while walking through a minefield

we are two peas in a pod
I wash her parents' dishes

vacuum their carpet
trying to make good impressions

it's not a perfect relationship
war movies versus French film
tofu or chocolate cake
I refer to her as my probable wife

we have finished graduate school
she is in New Mexico
I am in California
she calls again
asking me to visit
she has a good job
she'll pay the fare

I find another excuse not to go
wanting to fill some gap before committing

going to New Mexico requires
imagining a life

we end the call
she says
I love you
I say the same with hollow words

I can't make a commitment
there is no future to make a commitment to

eventually she gives up
she marries
my grief understands

she wants a family
she wants a life
she can imagine a future

GLIOBLASTOMA MULTIFORM STAGE FOUR

Visiting a childhood friend
he has just become a member of the club
first thing he says
I'm sorry, I never knew

his lesion is far more aggressive
chemo and radiation are working for now
a time of reprieve
his life hovering over his wife and boys

he takes them to the Grand Canyon
creating memories
while his shaved head looks cool

thankfully, he is unchanged
and we have the same discussions

before all this
he made a sharp turn to the right

I would try to change his mind
explaining this and that

now I just listen

RIVERS AND DAMS

Waiting to face the judge
she will demand

why can't you work

to answer
I must look her
and reality
in the eye

reluctantly
jettison my facades
dreams of normalcy
and concede

I have a rattled brain

confusion
absence
anxiety
fear
trauma
fanciful images and sounds

now I must sing to you
songs of loss and consequence
and stolen chunks of life

sensorineural hearing loss
broken lines of communication
and alienation

second percentile processing speed
I am slow

forgetful
neglecting to turn off the stove

migraine aura and sick headaches
sudden destructions of everyday life

diplopia scotomas and retinopathy
a two-dimensional world
with missing parts and colors

I will have to tell the judge
about the boss who barked

I'm lighting a fire under your butt
you have to work faster

for decades
I have labored to keep these in a box
keep that smile on my face

but the specter of the judge
permits no lies

farewell illusions and masks
you served me well

now
grief
terror
rage
flow like a river

now I must honestly address
friends and family

in the nauseating language
of intracranial destruction
and declare my deficits

my choice to be stoic
not weep and tremble
rendered obsolete

tears stream
my face quivers
as bits of truth fly free

no your honor
this is not the life I sought

no your honor
I can't compete in the stampede

no your honor
exposing my foibles and scars
is not a clever trick

no your honor
I try to get up each morning
put on a smile
and keep building these mighty dams

behind which
I can swim
in Lake Happy Face

the fees paid
in the pain and torments
of dissimulation

so maybe the judge is doing me a favor
yanking my finger
out of my dike
and letting the river flow

better than dog paddling
behind those dams I built
that burst

now the river flows
carrying with it
melancholy
anxiety
ruminations and limitations

and perhaps
mygraine

Mom used to tell me
laugh and the world laughs with you
cry and you cry alone

your honor
before you
I stand naked

and for a moment
wash away those fabrications
calm those locks and inflammations
sleep through the night
tame the scintillations
let my spirit go where it will
a genuine expression
on my face

MIGRAINE AS A VOICE

22 February 2014
1:00 PM

driving to university
word processor and printer
to work on memoir

oh shit

aura
vision fading quickly
standard three choices

abort and try to get home
before I can't see

call for someone
to rescue me

sit in the car
hope it will stop
and not become

full blown
six hour
incapacitating
agonizing pain

I try something new
pull car over in quiet shade
and ask

what do you want

BE TRUTHFUL AND DO A GOOD JOB OF IT

he is loud
angry
grizzly voiced
a mature man
impatient
and frustrated with me

who are you
I ask

WHO YOU MIGHT HAVE BEEN

the aura suddenly halts
I can see clearly

what do you want
I ask

no response
but I know his thoughts

a short visit
like Marley's ghost
his demands

stop lying
stop pretending
stop avoiding
stop procrastinating

stop waiting for nirvana
to arrive by itself

accept yourself
put yourself back together again
and live

THE SOUNDS OF MADNESS

It's noisy tonight
that sprinkler
bup bup bup bup bup bup bup bup bup bup bup bupping
incessantly
in my right ear

the roaring vacuum cleaner
MMMMMMMMMMMMMMMMMMMMMMMMMM
MMMMMMMMMMMMMMMMMMMMMMMMMM

and the midbrain hissing
ssssssssssssssssssssssssssssssssssssssssssssssss
ssssssssssssssssssssssssssssssssssssssssssss

like the bursting gaskets
in those submarine movies

I can put up with you
most of the time
ignore it by day
then drift off to fitful sleep

it's you motley groups
of mangled cilia

lost that sensorineural day
that rattle me

wailing in scattered pure tones
A's B's C's D's E's F's G's
flats sharps majors minors

in broken blocks of language
you gossip and sing incoherently

agrzhabrishtwlsjrowh dhoseksxhsxh jjwwythfjghvsoer dhasoe hsz
ppolkjmghrifubngkfelmcvxgiklgjewsvcxkjophgnbmfjrgkhjbfjdvnbtyx

I've had to work hard
to tolerate your bantering

but I hit the panic button
when you find a place in our cerebrum
that fashions your gibberish
into the words of ghosts

like that desperate voice
slowly counting

forty-one
forty -two
forty-three
forty-four

and the shrill
Jacob Marley
who demanded

WHAT WILL AN OLD SCHOOLBOY DO

when you make such alarming talk
I might take pills
in an off-label way
send you back to your fox holes

and leave me alone
with the sprinkler and the vacuum cleaner
who make a racket
but have nothing to say

TWO FRIENDS, MY DOCTOR AND YOSEMITE

Sixteen years post Seventeen
Blake, Jeff and I
planning what will be
an ambitious Yosemite adventure

am I up to
backpacking into the wilderness?

resolve determination and perseverance
good words to have in your backpack

as well as
two strong lifelong friends

we find a beautiful spot to camp
beside a waterfall
and its river

I build my best campfire

we make grilled cheese sandwiches
and tell stories late into the night

Blake scares off a bear
intent on breaking the tree branch
from which hang our packs and food

Jeff begins drawing this
landscape
which now hangs from my wall

 yet this experience was almost aborted
the day before setting out

crackling noises
emanating from beneath my scalp
shunt catheter disintegrating

I call Dr. G
should I cancel the trip
and come in tomorrow

he says
can you come now

arriving at the neurosurgery department
the lights are dim

the outpatient staff gone
departed for the day

walking quickly to the front desk
Dr. G processes
my Kaiser card

fills out forms
checking me in himself

how's your Mom
he asks

at ease as a receptionist
he returns to the role of family neurosurgeon

examining shunt catheter and valve
checking for signs
of trouble

satisfied there is no danger
he wishes me a good trip

how clear it is
he wants me to walk through the mountains

how clear it is
he wants me to enjoy myself

how clear it is
he wants me to live my life

SHERPAS OF THE MIND

Age fifty-five
Matt and I stop short of Oat Mountain's summit
but are treated to
an expansive view of the San Fernando Valley
where I grew up
and still live

I've tried to reach that pinnacle many times
but always fall short

at age sixteen
attempting to reach the top

Blake and I
failed to preconceive
the numerous foothills
blocking our path

finally reaching a patch of ice
we threw snowballs at each other
and called it a day

after that roads were opened
the hike up became shorter
though my path became quite rocky

but even so
many advisors
sages, healers and guides

enabled Seventeen and I
to arise from our setbacks
surmount those hills

and shout out that day with Matt
to the world below

I had post-traumatic stress!

I have had depression!

I have generalized anxiety disorder!

Seventeen emerged knowing
nothing of the brain
or diseases of its mind

and acquainted with
but a handful of mythical
therapists

Lucy Van Pelt
Sidney Freedman
Bob Hartley

in the time of his affliction
after each bombshell and setback

Seventeen got up
and marched on smiling

but when the good news came
tumor gone
treatment over

no battles to confront
no more fans cheering him on

there appeared
unlabeled
unaddressed
explosive

feelings

uncertainty
anxiety
terror
rage

his compass
silently spinning

one thing certain
he dreaded that dangling label

mental illness

must be silent and strong
no weakness allowed

but awareness emerged
something has slipped out of control
he can't climb this mountain
by himself

conceding
he consults Dr. G
who explains

psychologists are trained to help with feelings

psychologists
feelings

stigma
stigma

dogs are trained
elephants are trained

if he's going to lie on somebody's couch
that someone should have god given natural ability

regardless
an appointment is made
to see Dr. J

who explains
a lot of raging water
under your bridge
now that you can slow down
feelings are catching up

when Seventeen states that he feels like
smashing things with a baseball bat

Dr. J says
we can arrange that
and there are pills that can help
or you can try these relaxation recordings
basic Buddhist stuff

Seventeen and the baseball bat
choose the recordings

breathing
muscle relaxation
visualization

Seventeen feels better
and as he prepares to leave
for university in New England

Dr. J sends him off with thumbs up
but Seventeen leaves the tapes at home

he wants to think
he has put out his fires

but he has only begun
to climb this mountain

four fun years of growth
healing and occasional migraines

end with graduation
and emotional crisis

Seventeen returns to California
knowing he still needs help
and has a lot of work to do

a social worker is recommended
Morrie is a good guy to talk to
wise and grandfatherly

helps Seventeen continue to loosen his bolts
shepherds him through another breakdown
and says

you are not crazy
broken or damaged
this seems par for the course
and presents an idea to chew on

instead of labeling an interest in the brain
and its malfunctions
as an unhealthy obsession

you can see it
as a way of mastering the trauma

that bulb above
Seventeen's head lights up
trauma!

yes, what happened was
traumatic

Seventeen is comfortable
climbing up this hill with Morrie
but this licensed clinical social worker
retires

after his next breakdown
Seventeen's Mom says

we're going to take care of this
once and for all
and Seventeen is brought to
a psychiatrist

Dr. A offers understanding and empathetic words
that fuse with the wisdom
given by the others

and sends Seventeen
satisfied and appreciative
back on the trail

at times
Seventeen will welcome
medication's ability
to keep him calm

but this is a rest stop
not ascension

over the following years
through his thirties, forties
and into his fifties

there are many foothills to climb
crevasses in which to fall

and more help from healers
therapists of all kinds

a psychologist will say
I'm raising my rates

medical social worker will cushion
a descent into migraine hell

a clinical social worker
will try EMDR

as always
two steps forward
one step back

Seventeen's Rabbi says
Nirvana is not what you think it is

shit will happen
and continue to happen
we learn how to deal with it

Seventeen continues to grapple
with his mountain

he wants a more
time tested
well-trodden
evidence based path
to deal with it

maybe he will become a therapist
so back to school

introductory psychology
biopsychology
abnormal psychology
nutrition and the brain
psychology and aging

we can help our sympathetic
and parasympathetic nervous systems
learn to live in harmony

to navigate
the raging currents
and still waters of life

that compassion and empathy
diet and exercise
are effective meds

and as in a song
Neil Young wrote for his wife
that love is a healer

he tells a neurology nurse about his anger
she says
read Thich Nhat Hanh

East meets West
Seventeen tells his allopathic family practice doc
I need someone who gets it

doc says
Kim gets it

first thoughts
regarding this marriage and family counselor

she is good-looking
wicked smart
funny and makes him laugh

they are kindred spirits
can talk about anything
he hopes she's single
he tells her

when my life seems like easy street

she answers

you feel as if danger is at your door

she will guide him
towards the Practice
books and teachers
mindfulness and meditation
across gorges and up to high places

family crises
compassion

nervous breakdown
sympathy

status migraine with aphasia
empathy

hearing loss
patience

disability battles
kindness

prostate cancer
acceptance

he is on the path
that summit still far off
but getting closer

and with each hill scaled
a superior view

THE PRACTICE MEANS PRACTICE

First challenge after cure
manage anxiety

Seventeen embraces medication at times
but wants to heal
rather than medicate

1980 psychologist gives him
1980 relaxation tapes

cosmic
not yet mainstream
potentially powerful

but are these mental exercises
transformative

Seventeen uses practices
occasionally
when in crisis
and suffering symptoms

he did not understand
if the goal is transformation
the Practice means practice

at thirty-one
Seventeen the struggling teaching assistant

parks his car a half hour before class
and visualizes himself

with great results
a calm and effective teacher

at forty-one
a nurse introduces him to Thich Nhat Hanh

and Seventeen
really begins to address his anger

to practice living in the moment
aware of what is happening

within him
and without him

and to start listening
to those authentic inner voices

at forty -five
amidst another breakdown

his public health cousin brings from the university
meditation CD's for a new millennium

Kim walks beside him
introduces him to some East – West amalgamators

he reads the Dali Llama
notes the similarities to Jewish ideas

Judaism says meditate upon this
be mindful of that

but lacks instruction
how to do this

over the years
through teachers and books

the practice and the science
begin to fuse

and Seventeen can talk to his doctors
without feeling silly

yes, Buddhist monks and western physicians
are falling in love

and as I arise from Seventeen
from skepticism and laziness

I can clearly see
that with commitment, faith and practice

as the science paralleling my experience
is telling me

we really can modify and reshape
our brains, attitudes
perceptions and behavior

★★★

they must stay down
they will stay down

I am breathing in
I am breathing out

I am breathing in
relax

I am breathing in
I am calm

I hear you my anger
I will take care of you

keep me on this path
I am breathing out

give me strength
I am breathing out

give me wisdom
breathing out

guard me from lashon rah (evil tongue)
breathing out

keep me from pouring fuel
on the fire

I can consider and respond
rather than react and scream

give me sympathy
I am not the center of the world

what is hateful to me
I shall not do onto others

love my neighbor
as myself

honor my mother
honor my father

if not now
when

THE GRATITUDE WINDOW

I return to the operating room
thirty-five years later a man
my aging shunt valve to be removed

uncomfortable
that device behind my ear
often painful and hard to sleep

now threatening to pierce my scalp
and infect my brain

it will be good to part with this once life preserving contraption
rest my head comfortably on a pillow
knowing my central nervous system can manage its own
    plumbing

still, shunts and cerebrospinal fluid are tricky
high pressure low pressure
infection hemorrhage

it will take three attempts
for my surgical team and I
to reach equilibrium

they've rebuilt this hospital
but I'm the one who's changed

back then Seventeen was
a terrified boy
trying to be brave

now with maturity
therapy, love and mindfullness meditation
gratitude has emerged

through the window of my new room
that same hazy view of Los Angeles
Sunset boulevard and the Church of Scientology

Seventeen looked out long ago musing
it's a big beautiful world
I want my part

he was returned to the world
growing up to see
some of its sorrows

how fortunate to be
attached to wires and tubes
in this new intensive care unit

the TV depicts the mayhem in Paris
as my young nurse
caresses my hands

she's not really caressing
rather searching for a good vein for an IV
but I pretend she's caressing

we discuss current events
and her career plans
she's studying to be a nurse practitioner

the orderly brings my breakfast
broccoli, sweet potato and green tea with honey

I've learned how to keep my postoperative digestive tract happy
have plenty of time to practice mindfulness meditation

you're looking good the doctor says
though I'm jobless and alone
you can go home in a few days

I look out the window
where would I be without all these people
a fine second life I've had

Amherst and Manhattan
coral reefs at Sharm el-Sheikh
and their lionfish, sharks and manta rays
the 1991 solar eclipse at Baja

we had a spontaneous picnic
family and friends on the beach at Bet Cherut
when my brother got married

and there have been many
romantic walks with women
that went nowhere

is there anything I should not do
I asked Dr. G after he installed the shunt
you shouldn't stand on your head

so I jumped off waterfalls in the Galil
walked the Yosemite high country with Jeff and Blake
flew with the seagulls at Torrey Pines in a kite

I am free of the illusion
that we take care of ourselves
by ourselves

thank you Mom, Dad, family, friends, healers and strangers
thank you MRI builders Dilantin factory workers
shunt valve manufacturers and affordable caregivers

the nurse takes me for a walk
we pass very ill people
they have lived long lives

I hope that they have worked and appreciated and loved
made other people happy been treated fairly
and passed through life without too much trouble

I say goodbye to my doctor
nurses
and the person who cleaned my room

my eighty year-old father
arrives in his aging Toyota
we roll along with the LA traffic

towards home on a darkening November afternoon
hoping my ventricles will remain content
and discussing the improvements made to the freeway

A FANCIFUL CONVERSATION WITH THE MINISTER OF MIGRAINE AURAS AND HEADACHES

Host: You've been overseeing auras and migraine headaches for David for almost forty years now. We can't cover every episode in your long relationship with him, maybe you can tell us about some of the significant events that parallel his development.

Minister: OK, so he's cured by radiation. The tumor is gone. He manages to complete all that missed schoolwork, graduate high school and goes on a one-year program to live and work on a kibbutz, a communal farm, in the desert in Israel.

Host: How was he doing so soon after all that trauma?

Minister: On one hand he's doing well. He's with people. He's working, rebuilding his strength, hiking and sightseeing. So, in a lot of ways he's healing. But on the other hand, he's not doing well at his work assignments. His deficits cause him problems which he doesn't want to confront. He has friends but his relationships with girls are kind of clinical. And, with a few exceptions, he doesn't talk about the previous year. He has no sense of a future or what he's going to do in college. He has a kind of day to day existence. The auras he experienced earlier continue and he's starting to experience headaches.

Host: How did he respond to that?

Minister: With frustration and a hope that it would just go away. That it's temporary and will stop.

Host: So David comes home and starts college at a local university. How does that proceed?

Minister: He begins having migraines on a regular basis. The headaches are coming every three months and they are very painful.

Host: What were they like?

Minister: In these early years, nausea would come and when he threw up, he would really wretch, as if he was trying to exorcise something. The toilet was like an altar and there was this violence as if he was trying to get something out of himself.

Host: Was he trying to get the trauma, the experience of the brain cancer out?

Minister: Perhaps. And he makes an interesting discovery. He's becoming aware of his anger. And an aura starts up. The usual pattern is that it starts as a point of flashing light that gradually enlarges then slowly subsides and is followed by pain. So as this aura is intensifying, he goes into his room, shuts the door and starts screaming and punching his pillow. And within seconds, the aura stops and disappears like turning off a switch.

Host: Wow, a cure perhaps?

Minister: No, not a cure. You can't yell and pound the walls if you're in school, at work, or on an airplane. And this is a physical way of discharging energy. This is not a way to come to terms with complex, difficult feelings.

Host: So how was this episode helpful?

Minister: He acknowledged that anger was a component of his life that he had to address.

Host: So what is happening in his life at this point?

Minister: He transfers to a university in New England. He follows a female friend's advice to join her there. He's happy with the school, he's in a college town and getting involved in campus life. He loves New England and the winters. And the two of them get quite close. But he knows this is a short-term escape.

Host: From the tumor?

Minister: Yes, but he is also very close to this young woman.

Host: Is this a potential relationship?

Minister: On one hand, yes, he is comfortable and they are a nice couple. On the other hand, there is the traumatized boy who needs to work through the anger and the need to be taken care of. And in regard to the latter, he is comfortable having painful migraines in her presence.

Host: How did she feel about this?

Minister: I don't know. I live in his head, not hers. But one can imagine that this might be something difficult, a heavy weight to deal with at this point in a relationship.

Host: He is not ready for a relationship that might lead to marriage.

Minister: No, and he is aware of this problem, but it is a deep secret he keeps to himself.

Host: And the migraines continue.

Minister: Yes.

Host: Is he able to graduate from college?

Minister: Yes, but he has no idea what to do with himself apart from keeping anxiety at bay. He would like to replicate the relatively calm undergraduate years so he returns to California and enrolls in a graduate program, a combination of anthropology and film. It's interesting and keeps him busy.

Host: One can be a lost soul starting out as an undergrad at eighteen years old and find their way. That's part of the college experience. But in grad school, one is expected to have an idea of why they are there and what their goals are.

Minister: David was of the mindset that if he kept kicking this can down the road, things would eventually fall into place. He still had a lot of growing up to do.

Host: How are his elders reacting to this?

Minister: A professor he is close to says to him, "It's nice to be in a graduate program and keep busy but it seems to me you haven't resolved your experience. You're still living at home. You probably want to get married and start a family, am I right?" His father cried out in worry and frustration, "We want you to have a life!"

Host: So how did migraine respond?

Minister: Now he was having cluster headaches. Cluster headaches are extremely painful and they keep coming back, one after the other, for days. David was taken to the emergency room where a physician erroneously determined that he had a recurrence of brain cancer. He collapsed into an intense state of anxiety, experiencing flashbacks and reliving his surgeries and hospitalizations.

Host: So, what happened after that?

Minister: He recovered, made up the assignments he had missed and got back into the groove of school.

Host: And he finishes the program, he graduates?

Minister: Yes, with perseverance, and encouragement from his teachers, he graduates. But that day another cluster headache struck, bringing a week of severe pain so distracting, he neglected to take his anticonvulsants and had a seizure. With that, came more flashbacks and grief. This was his fraught matriculation from graduate school.

Host: What may have been behind the unleashing of all that havoc?

Minister: Perhaps rage related to the brain illness, the fear of seizures, of losing control; of his brain running wild. But also, there was the struggle to grow up and create a life. Face your demons. You can't keep plodding along forever.

Host: What happens now?

Minister: Well, his mom takes him to see a psychiatrist. And the doctor says, "If I just graduated, didn't have a job, had a terrible migraine and a seizure, I'd be depressed too." And the doctor's understanding comment puts things in perspective and validates David's feelings. And he gets into his pick-yourself-up mode. His parents are supportive. He has a place to live. He has his friends. And the migraines will, perhaps let's say, hibernate for a while.

Host: Is he discussing any of these events with his friends?

Minister: No, maybe it's too painful to discuss. Maybe he doesn't want to change the image he thinks they have of him. Healed from the illness. Same old Dave. Even though he is not.

Host: But he moves on.

Minister: Yes, he sets his sights on moving forward. He finds part-time jobs. He takes journalism classes at the community college and quickly becomes a star writer for their newspaper.

Host: Where does he go with that?

Minister: Well, he really enjoys this. He wins awards, and the instructors want him to continue as an editor but he doesn't take the offer. Maybe it's that fear of commitment. Maybe he doesn't think he can handle it. It's hard to understand him at times. But after a while, a friend from grad school helps him get a part-time job on a prominent television documentary.

Host: So how does he do at this job?

Minister: It's a documentary about World War One. He does research pertaining to the Armenian genocide. He gets satisfaction contributing to the project, likes the work and is excited getting up in the morning.

Host: So, is he starting, perhaps, to launch a career that gives him satisfaction that he might succeed at?

Minister: Perhaps.

Host: Does his health affect his ability to work?

Minister: Well, he's working part-time, not at a full production pace with deadlines and all that pressure. So, although the illness has made him slower and affected his ability to multi-task, he's kind of in a sweet spot. That is, his assignments are coming one at a time, he's not being pressured. He can take his time, focus on what he's doing and turn in good results.

Host: And what about the auras and headaches?

Minister: He's not experiencing auras and headaches.

Host : So where do things go with this job?

Minister: The job ends well and he's hired by an international project which is recording oral histories of Holocaust survivors.

Host: Considering everything David has been through, wasn't it difficult for him to listen to those terrible stories?

Minister: He's very good with these subjects. He handles them well.

Host: So how does this experience work out for him?

Minister: On one hand he's working full time and earning a living. He finds the work meaningful and gets along well with his co-workers. He moves into an apartment. He travels and even tries something he always wanted to do, hang gliding. On the other hand, red flags are popping up. His disabilities affect his ability to keep up with the production pace. He's expected to finish two assignments a week but barely completes one. His boss warns him, "I'm lighting a fire under your butt. You've got to speed up!" The quality of his work, however, is good, so the threats are never carried out. But he's always under that pressure.

Host: Why doesn't he discuss his disabilities with his employer?

Minister: Where does he start? Which problems does he try to explain first; processing speed, short term memory, vision, hearing, multitasking? And he is still doing a fairly good job of compensating for them.

Host: And how is he getting along with people, his social life?

Minister: Well, that's another red flag. He's socializing with women, but it's like a game to him, he's not taking things seriously.

Host: He's afraid of intimacy, of commitment?

Minister: Yes, he enjoys socializing but he can't discuss his experiences, his deficits, his fear that he might not be able to be a good provider. And he worries about fathering children, that he might be carrying bad genes, brain tumor genes.

Host: So the opportunities are there but he never develops any relationships.

Minister: He does develop a relationship with a woman whose company he enjoys but with whom he has limited interest. She, on the other hand, is in love with him and wants to marry him. The idea of marriage is totally beyond him but he feeds on her attention, and so goes along with it, a romantic relationship, telling himself it's good practice. Well, of course this behavior is insensitive, immature, and hurtful. But he plays this game. And they have this closeness and he begins to let a few things out. And she responds by saying things to him that while harsh, are insightful and he knows carry a bit of truth.

Host: What does she tell him?

Minister: "You are very immature, you are a little boy, you are so needy." And when he attempts to explain and talk about the darker parts of his life, she says impatiently, "I'm your girlfriend, not your psychologist!" And that sounds insensitive, but it doesn't really bother him because he knows there's some truth to it. And you can see, perhaps that's why he's been in the habit of keeping things to himself.

Host: So that relationship, I assume, didn't last very long.

Minister: No, and soon after that he found another job which would have different lessons.

Host: Please tell us about that.

Minister: Well, some of his previous employers are starting a new project about the history of the Jews. They hire David to do the research for it; they were impressed by his previous work.

Host: Sounds like a big step forward for him.

Minister: Yes, it's a lot of responsibility and it allows to him to really plough into this subject, consulting rabbis and scholars. He really has to apply himself.

Host: He's moving along with his life.

Minister: Yes, he has a sense of growing as a person. He's thinking, this might be it; I'm going to make it in the world.

Host: So how do things progress?

Minister: Unfortunately, problems start to occur almost as soon as he starts.

Host: But everything seems to have started so well.

Minister: David did not have a good sense of how to function in the working world. He still hasn't matured into some aspects of adult life; what it means to be hired to do a job, the politics and pressures of the workplace. He wants to do a good job, but he can't walk that tightrope between doing what he thinks is right and stepping on people's toes.

Host: So how did this experience pan out regarding his career?

Minister: The project came to an end, and that employer wasn't going to work with him again. This is a hard field to break into, even for someone without David's limitations.

Host: He has been migraine free for a while, hasn't he?

Minister: Yes, he has been free of migraine for nine years. He believes they are gone forever. He's made a lot of progress and has been able to take care of himself financially. But he knows that he wasn't able to make the best of a good opportunity, that he is in a field in which it is very difficult to succeed. And so his sense that his life is going to fall into place begins to disintegrate.

Host: So how does David adapt?

Minister: An interesting episode occurs at this time as his streak of employment and good luck ends. He's in a store and a song comes on over the loudspeaker. It's a song about memory and change, and David is listening and tears start streaming.

Host: Why did the song touch him like that?

Minister: It struck me that for the first time, David was acknowledging that the changes that had come in his life, to his body, to his brain, might make it more difficult, despite all that perseverance, to have that expected model life.

Host: That life being?

Minister: A stable job, a family, two kids and a dog. Along that line to some extent. But also, a life in which the brain cancer had been a bad episode that could be overcome without any significant negative changes, long term effects, or consequences.

Host: So, he accepts the changes and plots another course?

Minister: He starts preparing to go back to school and retrain for another career.

Host: Is that just running away again?

Minister: Well, this time he's thinking hard about an appropriate career path.

Host: So what is he thinking of, what is he studying?

Minister: He's thinking about psychology and mental health. He has, for obvious reasons, developed an interest in the brain, and he likes listening and talking to other people about their struggles. So he starts preparing for the entrance exams and taking prerequisite courses. A lot of work but it keeps him busy.

Host: And how are the migraines, it has been ten years without migraines?

Minister: At this point he starts having them again. Mostly short, mild auras about once a month. Annoying but not debilitating at first. But they will worsen.

Host: What happens?

Minister: Well, his mother becomes very ill, requiring months of treatment to resolve. And so there is a lot of work regarding hospitalization, rehabilitation and caretaking.

Host: So how does David handle all this?

Minister: He takes on a lot of the work and stress, interacting with doctors, nurses, therapists, insurance, and caretakers.

Host: That sounds like a lot to take on.

Minister: Yes, and in some ways it becomes a personal crusade for him. On one level, his own experience gives him a lot of empathy; he relates to his mother's fear and discomfort. He also has a very complicated sense of guilt, tied to a belief that his own health issues weigh heavily on his parents, especially his mom.

Host: So he's working extra hard to mitigate her suffering.

Minister: Beyond what most people can take on in a healthy way. A few months later he has a migraine and loses his ability to speak. He is admitted to the hospital. He is aware that the doctors are unsure what's going on. They are looking for tumors, blood clots, hemorrhages, infections. His mind is in a fog, a swirling state of auras and aphasia that will continue for days.

Host: What was he experiencing?

Minister: It's like being underwater. His sister and cousins are with him. They look familiar, but he's not sure who they are. He looks at a clock, but the numbers and hands appear to be broken and in the wrong positions. His universe has become the hospital bed.

Host: How is this episode resolved?

Minister: After ten days, his mind clears, his ability to speak returns, and the neurologists send him home with the label, "status migraine with aphasia," one doctor adding that, "you may have had what we used to call a nervous breakdown."

Host: But he picks himself up again.

Minister: Well, after all this, he recognizes that he needs help. Friends, family and therapists urge him to apply for disability assistance. So he applies to the California Department of Rehabilitation to help him find a job. They determine he is unable to work and that they can't help. He also applies for Social Security disability insurance and they tell him, "we think you can work, go find a job."

Host: So what does he do given this situation?

Minister: He is frustrated and reverts to that "I'll show you!" mode and applies to a professional program.

Host: What is he going to study this time? What's his plan?

Minister: He wants a job with stability and benefits. So he looks at several health professions and chooses a nearby program in gerontology.

Host: What does he see in gerontology?

Minister: He's had a challenging experience with his mother, so there's a personal element in that he'll have better skills. The school is promising jobs. So he goes through it thinking I'll just plug along and hopefully something will pop up.

Host: How are the migraines during this time?

Minister: He's having them every few weeks. He has several on the bus to school and during class. But soon, an event will occur that will really change things.

Host: What happens now?

Minister: He awakens one morning with very loud tinnitus in his left ear. It is an episode of sensorineural hearing loss. He is given steroids to try to restore his hearing but they have no effect. Within a few days he is completely deaf in that ear. And the steroids set off an attack of retinopathy which further diminishes vision in his right eye. In less than a week he is now partially deaf with further impairment to his vision.

Host: Is he able to continue with school?

Minister: He has a very supportive therapist who encourages him to continue, His teachers are helpful and he manages to graduate. But you don't get that kind of slack in the working world. It's much harder for him to work. And when he applies for jobs, he is told that he's not suitable.

Host: This must be so frustrating, he's tried so hard.

Minister: He tried, and for a long time it worked. Just keep pushing, don't complain, and try to do good work. But when you can't communicate with your boss, you can't follow directions, or forget them altogether, when you are working so slowly and carefully, one thing at a time, and you're worrying about the next migraine, you have to take an honest look at yourself and accept what has become beyond your ability.

Host: So what does he do?

Minister: Well, regarding the migraines, he works with his doctors and therapists, and makes a very concerted effort to find ways to calm his brain. And he does this with meditation and mindfulness and simultaneously finding dietary ways to calm the brain. And these practices will improve his life in many ways.

Host: And what about work?

Minister: He begins to concede that he can't maintain a standard, full-time job. He's going to need financial assistance. So he begins a long and humiliating process of applying again for Social Security Disability Insurance.

Host: But what is he going to do with himself? Who does he want to become?

Minister: There may be a silver lining here. Soon after losing his hearing he begins a class. He tells the professor, a psychologist, that he has hearing and visual deficits and is going to need help. The professor asks him if he knew the cause, and he tells her that he had brain cancer thirty years ago. Astonished, she states that she has never encountered a pediatric brain tumor survivor who has reached the age of forty-eight with the ability to be working on a second master's degree. "This story has to be told," she tells him.

Host: So David starts writing. How have his headaches and auras been during this period?

Minister: Well, he was driving recently and an aura began. He pulled over to the side of the road hoping that it would not evolve into a headache. After parking the car, he called out to whatever had launched this migraine beseeching it to answer his question, "What do you want from me!" A voice inside of him answered, "Take this work seriously and do a good job on it!" The scintillations stopped suddenly and his vision cleared.

THE BIRTHDAY PRESENT

Off to the bookstore
to buy a gift for my dying friend

I roam the aisles
knowing all his passions

he's still an armchair general
still loves the Beatles
Tolkien

and lately
The Game of Thrones

at nine he taught me how to play chess
he's raised two good boys

now the flow of magic poison
must stop
his body no longer capable of being
a battlefield

so many books and toys here
time to let go
of surprises and wrapping paper

I'll just call
and ask him what he wants

SURVIVORS AND COMPANIONS

In 1999 I moved into a single apartment
in Pico-Robertson, Los Angeles
home to many survivors

the landlords, husband and wife
had both been through it

the wife was mean, stingy and fought for every nickel
who knows what kind of hell she had been through

the husband was a nice guy
but I guess he had gotten used to rats
they didn't seem to bother him

to spruce things up
I bought Zamiaculcus zamiafolia
a new African exotic from the Congo

Zz had been living at M Forman Pottery and Plants Nursery
founded in 1946
after M Forman came back from The Navy and the War

she is extraordinary
turning eyes and making people say things

every few months
she launches a new stem
old stems turn brown, die and fall away
but leave a stump which stays alive and green

in the apartment Zz faced the TV
listened with me to famous people
and watched the towers fall

I've had jobs
good times and bad
friends have come and gone
but Zz always got her water

after the crash of 2008
I moved back in with Mom and Dad

Zz came along
seated in the back of my Civic

I said goodbye to M Forman and the Landlords
but sometimes regret not asking them
about before 1946
I suspect I won't be seeing them again

Zz keeps living in her pot
and never says a word

DER MENSCH TRACHT UND GOTT LACHT
(a person tries and God laughs)

My fifty-fifth year
the brain tumor experience out of my head
and onto paper

submitting queries
to publishers and literary agents

perhaps now it is behind me
I allow myself to dream

maybe
the book will be published

maybe
it will be well-received

maybe
I'll teach writing as healing

maybe
it will speak to a woman
with similar experience

for a few days
I am light and unencumbered

for a few nights
I sleep well

for a few days
I float in my imagination

I visit the doctor
some routine blood tests
he calls back

you have an aggressive form of prostate cancer

surgery
impotence
radiation
uncertainty

my literary queries generate
a growing pile of rejection letters

der mensch tracht und Gott lacht

ACKNOWLEDGEMENTS

Liz Zelinski made this project happen assigning me to create a memoir saying, "This story needs to be told."

Kizer Walker helped me to navigate a complicated publishing terrain and ultimately to find the right self-publishing option.

Maria Oparnica Simic nurtured my ability to write, critiqued the manuscript several times, gave me good books to read and lots of good advice – especially about maintaining a proper attitude regarding art and the marketplace.

Andrei Simic mentored me for three decades through my education, life, projects, work and finally, this account.

Ruth Rakoff inspired me by writing about her own experience with cancer. She gave me great advice: "Just start writing and you'll be surprised at what comes out." When it was done she critiqued and helped reshape it.

Cynthia Newhall read what I was writing, bounced around ideas with me, and constantly encouraged me saying, "Did you think this was going to be easy?"

Peter Murphy critiqued the manuscript, helped me improve it and guided me into the publishing world while at the same time helping me maintain a proper perspective regarding the art of writing.

Kim Kmetz helped me to reshape my thinking, alter my perspectives for the better and embrace life.

Patty Hausen got this project started and ignited my ability to write about difficult things by taking an interest in my life, interviewing family and friends who witnessed and shared my experience, and sharing her own poetry with me.

Susan Schwalb Gerson shared part of this trauma all those years ago, maintained an interest in this project and urged me to continue writing and allow myself the time I needed.

My mother suggested early on to "put it on paper." Much of this experience, in one way or another, has also been that of my parents, sister and brother. Their love and support has been the foundation of my life.

Made in the USA
Middletown, DE
09 April 2023

28538647R00139